Human Resources for Health

Overcoming the crisis

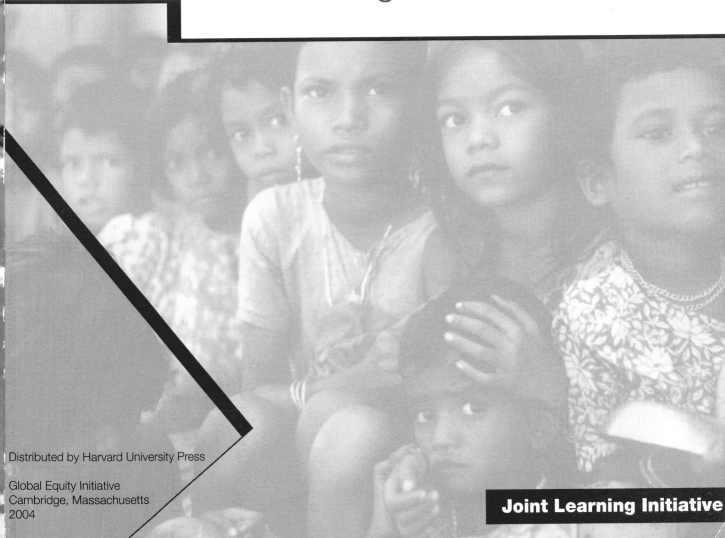

Distributed by Harvard University Press

Global Equity Initiative
Cambridge, Massachusetts
2004

Joint Learning Initiative

The Joint Learning Initiative (JLI), a network of global health leaders, was launched by the Rockefeller Foundation and was supported by a secretariat at Harvard University's Global Equity Initiative (GEI). The JLI acknowledges the generous financial support of the Rockefeller Foundation, Swedish Sida, the Bill & Melinda Gates Foundation, the Atlantic Philanthropies, and the World Health Organization in the production of this report. The responsibility for the contents and recommendations of the report rests solely with the leadership of the JLI, with Harvard University's GEI assuming ultimate technical and corporate responsibility.

 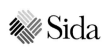 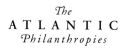 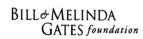

World Health Organization

Photo credits: Cover, title page, and pages 39, 40, 99, and 100, Lincoln C. Chen; pages 11 and 12, Jacob Silberberg/ Panos Pictures; pages 63, 64, 131, and 132, Carol Kotilainen.

Editing, design, and production by Communications Development Incorporated in Washington, D.C., with art direction by its U.K. partner, Grundy Northedge.

Human Resources for Health

Overcoming the crisis

Joint Learning Initiative

Contents

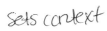

sets context

Tables

Preface

This report presents the findings and recommendations of the Joint Learning Initiative (JLI), an enterprise engaging more than 100 global health leaders in landscaping human resources for health and in identifying strategies to strengthen the workforce of health systems. Why did we embark on this journey? What was our destination? And what did we do along the way?

The JLI was launched because many of us believed that the most critical factor driving health system performance, the health worker, was neglected and overlooked. At a time of opportunity to redress outstanding health challenges, there is a growing awareness that human resources rank consistently among the most important system barriers to progress. Paradoxically, in countries of greatest need, the workforce is under "attack" from a combination of unsafe and unsupportive working conditions and workers departing for greener pastures. While more money and drugs are being mobilized, the human foundation for all health action, the workforce, remains under-recognized and under-appreciated.

To address this gap, the JLI was designed as a learning exercise to understand and propose strategies for workforce development. Seven working groups were established: supply, demand, priority diseases, innovations, Africa, history, and coordination. The open, collaborative, and decentralized design enabled each autonomous working group to draw the best from its diverse membership. Working groups were encouraged to ask tough questions, bring new ideas to the surface, and foster creativity and innovation.

The JLI's work was conducted in three phases. In a planning phase in 2002, leaders were recruited, a program framework was developed, and the work agenda was planned. 2003 was devoted to literature reviews, research, and consultations. More than 50 papers, many cited in this report, were commissioned, and more than 30 consultations were conducted around the world. These consultations engaged partner organizations and provided opportunities for us to listen to the voices of the health workers themselves. A third phase in 2004 focused on analyses and distilling lessons to generate the evidence base for the advocacy and dissemination of the JLI's findings and recommendations.

The JLI benefited from a truly unique combination of participation and leadership. Our co-chairs and members all volunteered their talents and time. Very importantly, an early priority was to achieve consensus that equity in global health would form the bedrock value for all JLI endeavors. This report thus represents not simply an analytical product but also an expression of our collective social commitment. As our interactions intensified over time, professional collegiality and personal friendships emerged. Even more important, mutual trust characterized our evolving relationships. This exceptional process was facilitated by the flexible financing provided by our core donors: the Rockefeller Foundation, the Swedish International Development Cooperation Agency (Sida), the Bill & Melinda Gates Foundation, and The Atlantic Philanthropies.

With the release of this report, the JLI has reached its destination. Given the challenges before us, completing this first leg simply launches us into the next phase of the journey. We in the JLI invite our colleagues and allies to join us on this road of strengthening human resources for health. Our hope is that this report, however modestly, illuminates the path ahead for us all.

Lincoln C. Chen
Co-chairs, JLI Coordination

Tim Evans

JLI Coordination working group members

Orvill Adams
Jo Ivey Boufford
Mushtaque Chowdhury
Marcos Cueto
Lola Dare
Gilles Dussault
Gijs Elzinga
Elizabeth Fee
Demissie Habte

Marian Jacobs
Joel Lamstein
Anders Nordstrom
Ariel Pablos-Mendez
William Pick
Nelson Sewankambo
Giorgio Solimano
Suwit Wibulpolprasert

JLI working group co-chairs

Coordination
Lincoln Chen, Harvard University, USA
Tim Evans, World Health Organization, Switzerland

Demand
Orvill Adams, World Health Organization, Switzerland
Suwit Wibulpolprasert, Ministry of Public Health, Thailand

Supply
Nelson Sewankambo, Makerere University, Uganda
Giorgio Solimano, University of Chile, Chile

Africa
Lola Dare, Center for Health Science Training, Research
    and Development International, Nigeria
Demissie Habte, BRAC School of Public Health, Bangladesh

Priority diseases
Mushtaque Chowdhury, BRAC, Bangladesh,
    and Columbia University, USA
Gijs Elzinga, National Institute of Public Health
and Environment, The Netherlands

Innovations
Jo Ivey Boufford, New York University, The Wagner School
    of Public Service, USA
Marian Jacobs, University of Cape Town, South Africa

History
Elizabeth Fee, National Library of Medicine: National Institutes
    of Health, USA
Marcos Cueto, Universidad Peruana Cayetano Heredia, Peru

Gender task force
Hilary Brown, World Health Organization, Switzerland
Laura Reichenbach, Harvard Center for Population
    and Development Studies, USA

Abbreviations

AIDS	Acquired immunodeficiency syndrome
CIDA	Canadian International Development Agency
DFID	Department for International Development, United Kingdom
DOTS	Directly observed treatment, short-course
FAIMER	Foundation for Advancement of International Medical Education and Research
G-8	Group of Eight
GAVI	The Global Alliance on Vaccines and Immunization
GDP	Gross domestic product
GNI	Gross national income
GTZ	Deutsche Gesellschaft für Technische Zusammenarbeit
HDI	Human development index
HIPC	Heavily indebted poor country
HIV	Human immunodeficiency virus
HRH	Human resources for health
ILO	International Labour Organization
IMF	International Monetary Fund
JLI	Joint Learning Initiative
MDGs	Millennium Development Goals
MTEF	Medium-term expenditure framework
NGO	Nongovernmental organization
ODA	Official development assistance
OECD	Organisation for Economic Co-operation and Development
OSI	Open Society Institute
PAHO	Pan American Health Organization
PEPFAR	President's Emergency Plan for AIDS Relief, United States
PPP	Purchasing power parity
PRSP	Poverty reduction strategy paper
SARS	Severe acute respiratory syndrome
SWAp	Sector-wide approach
TB	Tuberculosis
UNESCO	United Nations Economic, Scientific and Cultural Organization
UNFPA	United Nations Population Fund
UNICEF	United Nations Children's Fund
WHO	World Health Organization

Executive Summary

After a century of the most spectacular health advances in human history, we confront unprecedented and interlocking health crises. Some of the world's poorest countries face rising death rates and plummeting life expectancy, even as global pandemics threaten us all. Human survival gains are being lost because of feeble national health systems. On the frontline of human survival, we see overburdened and overstressed health workers—too few in number, without the support they so badly need—losing the fight. Many are collapsing under the strain. Many are dying, especially from AIDS. And many are seeking a better life and more rewarding work by departing for richer countries.

Today's dramatic health reversals risk more than human survival in the poorest countries—they threaten health, development, and security in an interdependent world. How the world community responds to these challenges will shape the course of global health for the entire 21st century.

The global health crisis occurs against a backdrop of mass poverty, uneven economic growth, and political instability. The vicious spiral of paralytic responses to threatening diseases is accelerated by three major forces assailing health workers.

- First is the devastation of HIV/AIDS—increasing workloads on health workers, exposing them to infection, and testing their morale. Many are becoming terminal care providers, not healers. Hardest hit are societies in sub-Saharan Africa, but the virus is also spreading rapidly from hot spots in Asia, the Americas, and eastern Europe.
- Second is accelerating labor migration, causing losses of nurses and doctors from countries that can least afford the "brain drain."
- Third is the legacy of chronic underinvestment in human resources. Two decades of economic and sectoral reform capped expenditures, froze recruitment and salaries, and restricted public budgets, depleting work environments of basic supplies, drugs, and facilities.

These forces have hit economically struggling and politically fragile countries the hardest.

> **We estimate the global health workforce at more than 100 million. Added to the 24 million doctors, nurses, and midwives that are routinely enumerated are at least three times more uncounted informal, traditional, community, and allied workers**

The power of the health worker

Even so, dedicated health workers across the world demonstrate commitment and purpose far beyond the call of duty. And their steadfast motivation is finally being matched by new political priorities and greater financial allocations for health—with the AIDS epidemic fueling public concern and social activism. Money—though still far from adequate—is beginning to flow, and some life-prolonging drugs are now far cheaper and more widely available than just a few years ago.

Accompanying these dynamics is the broader development compact forged by the United Nations (UN) to reach the Millennium Development Goals (MDGs) by 2015. These global goals, prominently featuring health, have become a focal point for rallying international cooperation to achieve time-bound targets. Emerging are many new programs, mechanisms, financing strategies, and actors.

To take advantage of these opportunities, a strong and vibrant health system is essential. Yet such systems are impossible without health workers who are the ultimate resource of health systems. Yes, money and drugs are needed, but these inputs demand an effective workforce. For it is people, not just vaccines and drugs, who prevent disease and administer cures. Workers are active, not passive, agents of health change. With their salaries often commanding two-thirds of health budgets, they weave together the many parts of health systems to spearhead the production of health.

Throughout history, periods of acceleration in health have been sparked by popular mobilization of workers in society. Higher worker density and better work quality—joining such social determinants of health as education, gender equality, and higher income—improve population-based health and human survival. The density of workers in a population can make an enormous difference in the effectiveness of MDG interventions to reach the MDGs. For example, the prospects for achieving 80 percent coverage of measles immunization and skilled attendants at birth are greatly enhanced where worker density exceeds 2.5 workers per 1,000 population. Seventy-five countries with 2.5 billion people are below this minimum threshold.

We estimate the global health workforce to be more than 100 million people. Added to the 24 million doctors, nurses, and midwives who are routinely enumerated are at least three times more uncounted informal, traditional, community, and allied workers. Those enumerated professionals are severely maldistributed. Sub-Saharan Africa has a tenth the nurses and doctors for its population that Europe has. Ethiopia has a fiftieth of the professionals for its population that Italy does.

With such wide variation, every country must devise a workforce strategy suited to its health needs and human assets. Here, we assign 186 countries to low, medium, and high worker density clusters (below 2.5, between 2.5 and 5.0, and above 5.0 workers per 1,000 population, respectively), with the low and high density clusters further sub-divided according to high and low under-five mortality. Among low-density countries, 45 are in the low-density-high-mortality cluster; these are predominantly sub-Saharan countries experiencing the double crisis of rising death rates and weak health systems. The remaining 30 low-density countries are mostly in Asia and Latin America, the predominant regions for the 42 moderate density countries. Among high-density countries, 34 are in the high-density-low-mortality

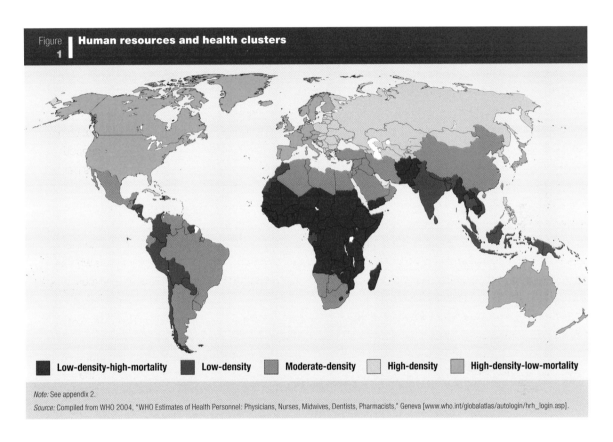

Figure 1 | Human resources and health clusters

Legend: ■ Low-density-high-mortality ■ Low-density ■ Moderate-density □ High-density ■ High-density-low-mortality

Note: See appendix 2.

Source: Compiled from WHO 2004, "WHO Estimates of Health Personnel: Physicians, Nurses, Midwives, Dentists, Pharmacists," Geneva [www.who.int/globalatlas/autologin/hrh_login.asp].

cluster, all wealthy countries, mostly members of the Organisation for Economic Co-operation and Development (OECD). The remaining 35 high-density countries are transitional economies or exporters of medical personnel.

All these countries, rich and poor, suffer from numeric, skill, and geographic imbalances in their workforce. And all countries can accelerate health gains by investing in and managing their health workforce more strategically. While maintaining a global perspective, we focus on low-density-high-mortality countries because of their dire health situations. For all countries, we conclude that our outstanding global challenges are:

Global shortages. There is a massive global shortage of health workers. Although imprecise quantitatively, we estimate the global shortage at more than four million workers. Sub-Saharan countries must nearly triple their current numbers of workers by adding the equivalent of one million workers through retention, recruitment, and training if they are to come close to approaching the MDGs for health.

Skill imbalances. Nearly all countries suffer from skill imbalances, creating huge inefficiencies. In some, the skill mix depends too much on doctors and specialists. In most, population-based public health is neglected. Many

3

countries must revamp their health plans toward a workforce that more closely reflects the health needs of their populations, especially by deploying auxiliary and community workers.

Maldistributions. Nearly all countries have maldistribution, which is worsened by unplanned migration. The urban concentration of workers is a problem everywhere. Improving within-country equity requires attracting health workers to rural and marginal communities—and retaining them. There is also a maldistribution between public and private sectors in many countries. And international equity is worsened by unplanned international migration, with the loss of nurses and doctors crippling health systems in many poor sending countries.

Poor work environments. Nearly all countries must improve work environments by scaling up good practices to strengthen the management of existing resources, assure adequate supplies and facilities, and create monetary and nonfinancial incentives to retain and motivate health workers. The voices of workers need to be heard.

Weak knowledge. The weak knowledge base on the health workforce hampers planning, policy development, and program operations. Information is sparse, data fragmentary, and research limited—deficiencies that must be remedied.

Workforce strategies

Evidence confirms that effective workforce strategies enhance the performance of health systems, even under difficult circumstances. Indeed, the only route to reaching the health MDGs is through the worker; there are no short-cuts. Workers, of course, are not panaceas. Building a high performance workforce demands hard, consistent, and sustained effort. For workers to be effective, they must have drugs and supplies. And for them to use these inputs efficiently, they must be motivated, skilled, and supported.

Appropriate workforce strategies can generate enormous efficiency gains. Successful strategies must be country-based and country-led, focusing on the frontlines in communities, backed by appropriate international reinforcement.

Community action, the focus of all strategies, should ensure access for every family to a motivated, skilled, and supported health worker. The base of the worker system consists of family members, relatives, and friends—an "invisible workforce," mostly female. They are backed by diverse informal and traditional healers, and in many settings by formal community workers. Beyond these frontline providers are doctors, nurses, midwives, professional associates, and nonmedical managers and workers who support effective practice. Although the national pattern of workers demonstrates extraordinary diversity, all strategies should seek to promote community engagement in recruiting and retaining workers and accounting for worker performance.

Country leadership and strategies are the leverage points for workforce development because governments set policies, secure financing, support education, operate the public sector, and regulate the private sector. Diverse national circumstances also mean that solutions must be crafted to unique country challenges.

❝❝ Managing the workforce for better performance brings together the health and educational sectors to achieve three core objectives—coverage, motivation, and competence

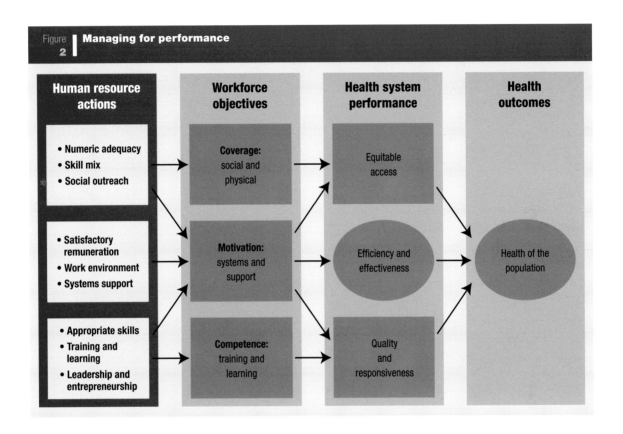

Figure 2 | **Managing for performance**

| **Human resource actions** | **Workforce objectives** | **Health system performance** | **Health outcomes** |

- Numeric adequacy
- Skill mix
- Social outreach

- Satisfactory remuneration
- Work environment
- Systems support

- Appropriate skills
- Training and learning
- Leadership and entrepreneurship

Coverage: social and physical

Motivation: systems and support

Competence: training and learning

Equitable access

Efficiency and effectiveness

Quality and responsiveness

Health of the population

But all country strategies should have five key dimensions—engaging leaders and stakeholders, planning human investments, managing for performance, developing enabling policies, and building capacity while monitoring results.

Workforce development is not merely a technical process—it is also political. It demands building a strong action coalition across all stakeholders with diverse interests. Health workers must be at the center, but collaboration must reach beyond the health sector to finance, education, and other ministries and beyond government to academic leaders, professional associations, labor unions, educational institutions, and nongovernmental

organizations. All must be involved in setting national goals, designing strategies, drawing up plans, and implementing policies and programs. Good data, invariably scarce where needed most, are essential to inform and guide such efforts.

Management of the workforce for better performance brings together the health and educational sectors to achieve three core objectives—coverage, motivation, and competence. Coverage strategies promote numeric adequacy, appropriate skill mixes, and outreach to vulnerable populations. Motivation strategies focus on adequate remuneration, a positive work environment, opportunities for career development, and supportive health systems. Competencies are advanced through educating for appropriate attitudes and skills, creating conditions for continuous learning, and cultivating leadership, entrepreneurship, and innovation. All these efforts should be oriented toward building national capacity. Progress and setbacks should be monitored for mid-course corrections.

Global responsibility must be shared because no country is an island in workforce development. Transnational flows of labor, knowledge, and financing imply that successful country strategies depend on appropriate international reinforcement. Some cross-border flows, left unattended, may generate negative health consequences—the "brain drain" from sending countries, for example. But properly harnessed, these flows have great potential—scaling up best practices and using foreign aid more efficiently are examples.

Critical is improving the management of transnational flows of highly skilled medical professionals. The migration of doctors and nurses resembles a "carousel" of multiple entry and exit paths—from low- to high-income regions. These migratory flows can produce many benefits—and generate much harm. Because blocking the movement of people violates human rights and is generally impossible to enforce, the global management of medical migration should seek to protect both health and human rights—dampening "push" forces by retaining talent in sending countries and reducing "pull" forces by aiming for educational self-sufficiency in destination countries. Global opportunities should be expanded by massively increasing educational investments in source countries and accelerating appropriate "reverse flows" of workers from better endowed to deficit countries.

The great potential for harnessing the transnational flow of knowledge for workforce development remains largely untapped. The diffusion of knowledge accounts for much of the spectacular health advances of the past century. Yet workforce data and research are sparse. Strategies must focus on bridging the knowledge-action gap, promoting the sharing of information, and strengthening the knowledge base. Especially important is inculcating a culture of research and promoting the diffusion of innovation among all countries.

After a decade of stagnation, official development assistance (ODA), another transnational flow of high potential, is finally turning around. We estimate that of a 2002 total ODA of $57 billion, 13 percent is directed at health—now increasing to about $10 billion. Most new funds are targeted at HIV/AIDS in sub-Saharan Africa. We also estimate that 30–50 percent, or about $4 billion of development assistance for health, is devoted to human resources—salaries, allowances, training, education, technical assistance, and capacity building. Applying $400 million of that to country strategies and capacities would reap enormous payoffs.

Current spending patterns on human resources are fragmented and inefficient. To invest more strategically, donor and policy coherence must be dramatically improved—changing attitudes about health workers as a crucial investment, harmonizing the workforce across competing categorical programs, and ensuring fiscal policies that support workforce improvements. For countries in a health emergency, international financial institutions must join in lifting public expenditure ceilings to permit donor support of the massive mobilization of the workforce that will be necessary.

ff **Applying $400 million to country strategy and capacity building would reap enormous payoffs**

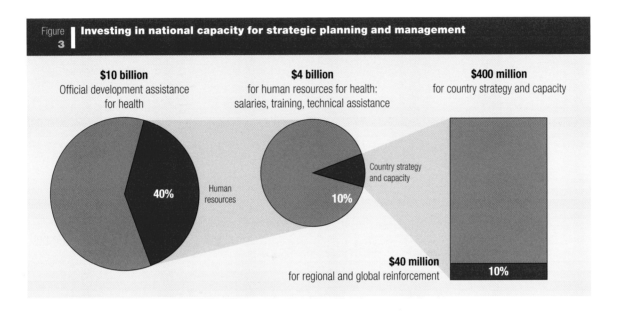

Figure 3 | **Investing in national capacity for strategic planning and management**

$10 billion
Official development assistance for health

40% — Human resources

$4 billion
for human resources for health: salaries, training, technical assistance

10% — Country strategy and capacity

$400 million
for country strategy and capacity

10%

$40 million
for regional and global reinforcement

Putting workers first

We call for immediate action to harness the power of health workers for global health equity and development. The imperative for action springs from the urgency of the health crisis, the timeliness of new opportunities, and the prospect that available knowledge, if applied vigorously, could save many lives. The cost of inaction is unmistakable—stark failures to achieve the MDGs, epidemics spiraling out of control, and the unnecessary loss of many lives. At stake is nothing less than the course of global health and development in the 21st century.

Urgency demands an exceptional response from the global community. At its core, the response must be country-based and country-led—because all global initiatives must be implemented, planned, and owned in specific national settings. That response must also be multidimensional. Technical approaches alone will not do, because adequate financing, strong leadership, and political

commitment are necessary. And the response must be inclusive, engaging all relevant stakeholders, including nonhealth and nongovernmental groups. In the poorest countries, that response must also include appropriate behavior by the international community, because external resources are needed to supplement domestic resources.

"Business as usual" will not do. The very credibility of national, regional, and global health institutions is under siege. Health emergencies, collapsing health systems, and crises in human resources cannot be sealed off to only the poorest countries. These global problems are ultimately shared. Strengthening the health workforce is a shared challenge that demands commonly developed solutions—a mutual responsibility of all. The key to unlocking our shared health future is to galvanize action by all actors to strengthen human resources for health—both to combat crises and to build sustainable systems.

7

> **Every country, poor or rich, should have a national workforce plan shaped to its situation and crafted to address its health needs**

Actions must be pursued over a "decade for human resources for health" (2006–2015) and implemented through action alliances. Crafting a workforce to meet national health needs requires sustained efforts over time—it cannot be a fleeting fad. This timeline also matches the remaining 10 years for achieving the MDGs. All agencies, training institutions, professional associations, nongovernmental bodies, and private initiatives should direct their efforts at a three-part agenda:

- Strengthening sustainable health systems in all countries.
- Mobilizing to combat health emergencies in crisis countries.
- Building the knowledge base for all.

Strengthening sustainable health systems

Every country, poor or rich, should have a national workforce plan shaped to its situation and crafted to address its health needs. These plans should aim to ensure access for every family to a motivated, skilled, and supported health worker. When feasible, that worker should be recruited from, accountable to, and supported to work in the community. Our specific recommendations:

- All countries should develop national workforce strategic plans to guide enhanced investments in human resources as the core component of strengthening national health systems.
- Academic leaders in educational institutions and health leaders in government ministries should engage in policy dialogues to develop an appropriate and effective national workforce, crafting health sector reform and shaping cadres of workers matched to priority national health needs.
- All countries should examine and increase their investments in appropriate education, deployment, and retention of human resources.
- An international regime should be crafted that recognizes the "exceptionalism" of medical migration, promoting the human right of free movement while protecting the health of vulnerable populations. We support national action in both sending and receiving countries, but not international "compensation" because of its infeasibility. Instead, we urge the launching of a global educational reinvestment fund in Southern countries—and sustainable "reverse flows" of diaspora, volunteers, and exchanges of workers, wherever appropriate.
- Global health and financial policymakers should work together to ensure an enabling fiscal environment for health workforce development. Donors should harmonize their investments to apply at least 10 percent or $400 million of their estimated $4 billion spending on human resources to strengthen strategic human capacities within countries. Of these national investments, 10 percent or $40 million should be earmarked for strengthening technical and policy cooperation on human resources at the regional and global levels.

Mobilizing to combat health emergencies

In countries severely affected by HIV/AIDS, especially those in much of sub-Saharan Africa, popular mobilization to harness workers is urgently required to

❝ In countries severely affected by HIV/AIDS, popular movements to mobilize health workers are urgently required to reverse the crisis of human survival

overcome the crisis of human survival. Crisis countries must assess the suitability of their current workforce and mobilize support for appropriate delegation of core health functions to well-trained community-based auxiliary workers. The support of donors, regional bodies, and global organizations is critical for effective implementation. Our specific recommendations:

- Urgently develop strategies to mobilize, retain, and train health workers to combat HIV/AIDS and other priority problems as part of strategies to steadily build primary health care systems. Sub-Saharan African countries should nearly triple the size of their workforces, adding the equivalent of one million workers, operating in work environments that enable them to be productive.

- Bring together country, regional, and global technical expertise on human resources for health through "virtual" and "operational" networks that can disseminate best practices and provide effective technical support to country-based and country-led actions.

- Create an enabling policy and financing environment by specifically ensuring supportive macroeconomic policies and the coherence of categorical funds for HIV/AIDS and other priority problems consistent with national workforce plans. Disease control programs should seek to achieve their priority targets while strengthening, not fragmenting, a sustainable workforce in the overall health system.

Building the knowledge base

Effective action, both urgent and sustained, requires solid information, reliable analyses, and a firm knowledge base. But data and research on human resources for health are underdeveloped, especially in low-density-high-mortality countries. National and global learning processes must be launched to rapidly build the knowledge base—essential for guiding, accelerating, and improving action. A culture of science-based knowledge building must be infused in the human resources community. Our specific recommendations:

- All countries should strengthen national data, information, analysis, and research in human resources for health. All workers should be counted and their social attributes and work functions should be collated to improve planning, policy, and programs.

- Research on workforce norms, standards, and best practices should be augmented, with the findings rapidly disseminated to improve workforce effectiveness in all countries.

- Funders, both national and international, should significantly enhance their investments in information and knowledge on human resources. In addition to strengthening country actions, these investments would provide a global public good.

Completing an unfinished agenda: Action and learning

Implementing this work agenda demands immediate action backed by simultaneous learning. We must spark a virtuous circle of acting, learning, adjusting, and growing—because we do not have all the answers and yet we must act urgently.

Because the key actions rest with national governments, we call on national leaders to implement these recommendations. We also call

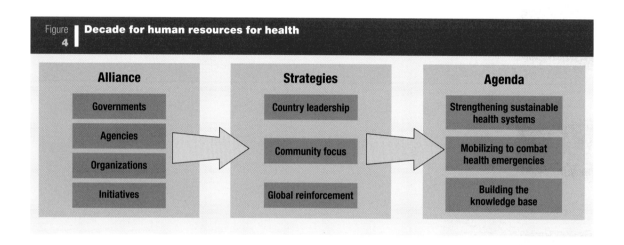

Figure 4 | **Decade for human resources for health**

Alliance
- Governments
- Agencies
- Organizations
- Initiatives

Strategies
- Country leadership
- Community focus
- Global reinforcement

Agenda
- Strengthening sustainable health systems
- Mobilizing to combat health emergencies
- Building the knowledge base

on international agencies—especially the WHO and the World Bank but also the UNDP, UNESCO, the Global Fund, the Global Alliance on Vaccines and Immunizations, the President's Emergency Plan for AIDS Relief, and others—to support coherent national action. Through collaborative planning and regular feedback, alliances for action can be systematically strengthened so that international actors play more effective roles in human resources for health at the country and community levels.

We also propose an independent, nongovernmental, five-year Action & Learning Initiative to take up the recommendations of the Joint Learning Initiative in advocacy, promoting shared learning, and monitoring progress. Operating through networks with nodes in the major world regions, the action-learning initiative will catalyze and reinforce global support of county action.

The advantage of an alliance for action is that most critical activities can be conducted by existing organizations without creating yet another cumbersome (and expensive) formal global program

or partnership. Success will depend, however, on how well existing institutions can ratchet up their capabilities and performance. Official agencies are urged to assume leadership roles in their respective areas of strength, while nongovernmental academia, professional associations, and social organizations are encouraged to join in this work, both directly and as facilitated by the Action & Learning Initiative.

*   *   *

It is impossible to underestimate the importance of a response to this call for action. At stake is nothing less than completing the unfinished agenda of the past century while addressing the unprecedented health challenges of this new century. Millions of people around the world are trapped in a vicious spiral of sickness and death. For them there is no tomorrow without action today. Yet much can be done through rapidly mobilizing the workforce and wisely investing to build a stronger human infrastructure for sustainable health systems. What we do—or fail to do—will shape the course of global health in the 21st century.

The Power of the
Health Worker

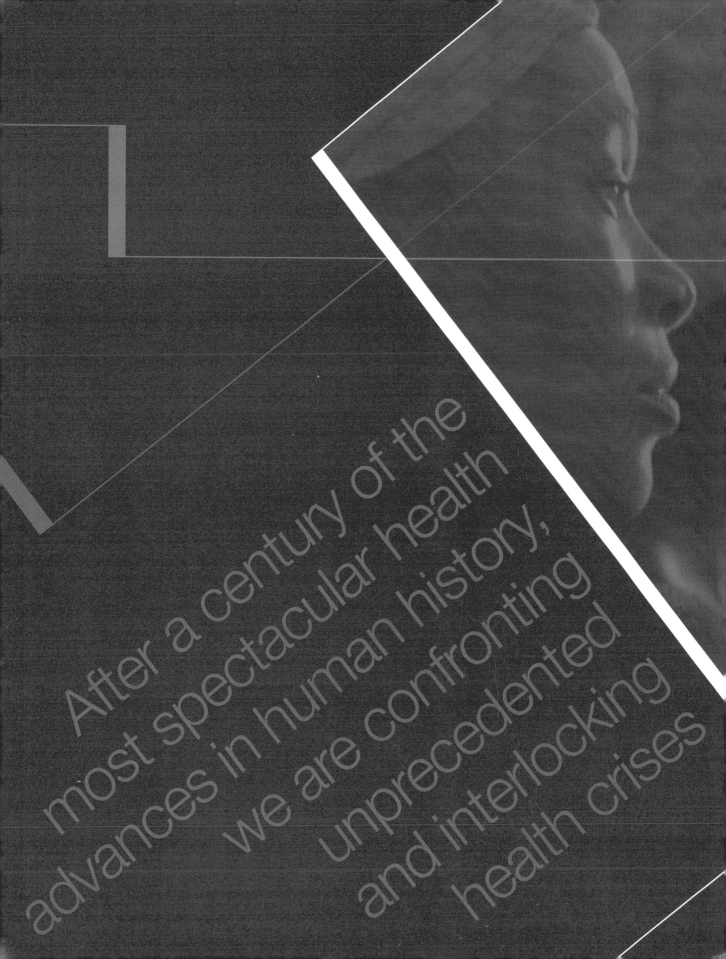

After a century of the most spectacular health advances in human history, we are confronting unprecedented and interlocking health crises

The Power of the Health Worker

After a century of the most spectacular health advances in human history, we are confronting unprecedented and interlocking health crises. We face rising death rates and plummeting life expectancy in some of the world's poorest countries, and new global pandemics that threaten us all. Human survival gains are being lost because extremely feeble national health systems are unable to cope and respond. Today's dramatic health reversals threaten not only human survival in affected countries but also development and security in an interdependent world. How the global community responds to these challenges will shape the course of global health for the entire 21st century.

People deliver health. It was investment in the world's health workers—from community workers and barefoot doctors to nurses and physicians—that made possible the science-based health revolution of the 20th century. Today's crisis reflects both new and resurgent diseases as well as neglect of human resources in the health sector, so critical for effective response. At the frontline of human survival in affected countries, we see overburdened and overstressed health workers, few in number and without the support they so badly need, losing the fight. Many are collapsing under the strain, many are dying, especially from AIDS, and above all, many are seeking a better life and a more rewarding work environment by leaving for richer countries.

Even so, dedicated health workers across the world demonstrate social commitment and purpose far beyond the call of duty. And their steadfast motivation is finally being matched by new political priorities and greater financial allocations for health— with the AIDS epidemic fueling public concern and social activism. Money—though still far from

❝ The promise will be realized only when the global community mobilizes and strengthens the power of the health worker

adequate—is beginning to flow, and life-prolonging drugs and technologies are now far cheaper and more widely available than just a few years ago. These initiatives hold much promise. But, this report argues, that promise will be realized only when the global community mobilizes and strengthens the power of the health worker, the most neglected yet most essential building block of effective health systems.

This chapter documents the forces that are decimating the health workforce in poor countries. Decades of neglect have relegated the health workforce to a policy backwater. The global labor market is drawing much-needed health workers from poor to rich countries. And the unique threat of HIV/AIDS is battering the health workforce in many countries. Tremendous opportunities are opening to act more effectively. But until now, a crucial element is missing: adequate investment in people.

This is the starting point for the Joint Learning Initiative (JLI), an independent network of more than 100 global health leaders from around the world. We began our inquiry by charting the composition of the global health workforce, its numbers, skills, and distribution. Next, we categorized countries into distinctive clusters to gauge how levels and patterns of health workers affect health outcomes. Finding remarkably little data on these important challenges, we commissioned research, with the findings presented here. This chapter concludes by pinpointing the major challenges for strengthening human resources for health, both globally and in countries in crisis.

Today's health crisis

History will applaud the 20th century for its remarkable achievements in human health. Our grandparents would never have dared dream about the pace of medical progress that nearly doubled life expectancy among the world's privileged, even surpassing the biblical three score years and ten. What made this possible? Advances in medical science and public health, along with better hygiene, higher income, improved nutrition, and socioeconomic developments—all combining to enable people to score victories over lethal pathogens.

Reflecting this upward trend of life expectancy, medical optimism dominated at mid-century. By the turn of the millennium, however, this confidence was rudely dashed by emerging and resurging health threats. The most notable: the HIV/AIDS pandemic, the biggest health catastrophe in human history. But an array of other communicable and noncommunicable killers also surged. Changing human ecology nurtured new pathogens, while globalization enabled familiar ones to threaten to spread in pandemic proportions. Among the conditioning factors: explosive urban growth, mass poverty, unprecedented international mobility, and intrusive human interactions with the environment. With our medical confidence deeply shaken, human fear has overtaken medical optimism.

Today's global health picture is one of great diversity, with life's chances and health's inequities sharply polarized. Poverty and inequality are both causes and symptoms of the crisis in health. Average life expectancy in many societies is less than half that of the privileged. And the gaps are widening. The wealthy continue to enjoy longevity up to and beyond 80 years, but life expectancy at birth is less than 40 in more than a dozen countries, nearly all in sub-Saharan Africa (figure 1.1). And hot spots of health's stagnation or reversal are found in all world

❝❝ Today's global health picture is one of great diversity, with life's chances and health's inequities sharply polarized

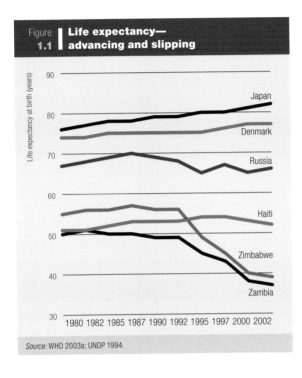

Figure 1.1 | Life expectancy— advancing and slipping

Life expectancy at birth (years)

Japan
Denmark
Russia
Haiti
Zimbabwe
Zambia

1980 1982 1985 1987 1990 1992 1995 1997 2000 2002

Source: WHO 2003a; UNDP 1994.

regions. These disparities are not just threats to global human security—they are moral and ethical affronts.

The HIV/AIDS pandemic is plunging sub-Saharan Africa into a profound crisis of survival. In countries severely hit, life expectancy is down sharply, and infant and child mortality is rising. Young women are dying in unprecedented numbers. Yet we are still in the early stages of this crisis. A decade after HIV prevalence climbs, AIDS deaths will rise, leading to a third wave of devastating societal impact—families dissolved, children orphaned, education and health disrupted, economic growth impeded, and political governance challenged. This is a confluence of unmitigated disaster without historical precedence. Already AIDS has increased hunger and food insecurity in Southern Africa.[1] In the worst scenarios, the very survival of people, nations, and civilizations is under siege.

Even as HIV/AIDS becomes the biggest killer in Africa, other diseases are emerging or resurging. Tuberculosis is gaining momentum among HIV-positive people with compromised immune defenses, and multidrug resistant strains are on the increase. Malaria, spreading widely, is also more resistant to today's treatments. Unless basic immunization is maintained, the common infectious diseases of childhood, already major killers, will resurge. Health crises are heightened by economic deprivation and political instability. Consider how humanitarian emergencies in the Democratic Republic of Congo, Liberia, Sierra Leone, Sudan, and Zimbabwe entrap populations in a vicious cycle with lethal combinations of violence, hunger, and disease.

Sub-Saharan Africa, the region hit hardest, will fall farther behind, and the widening international health gap will create a global health apartheid that is unsustainable, epidemiologically and morally. Nor are other world regions immune from health catastrophes. Russia and the former Soviet Union states are seeing reversals of life expectancy among adult men because of injury, alcohol abuse, and environmental hazards. Eastern European countries have the world's fastest growing HIV rates, driven largely by intravenous drug abuse. Countries in the Americas have largely escaped health crises—yet there are such exceptions as Haiti, with its crushing poverty, political instability, and high HIV rates. And there is cause for alarm in Asia, the world's most populous region. Unless there is immediate and effective action, India and China will soon be epicenters of the world's largest HIV epidemics.

Anticipating and reversing these health crises require a strong health system able to prevent and treat disease and promote good health. Yet,

" Advocacy has pushed global health onto the agenda of high politics

it is precisely where health crises are most severe that health systems are weakest—failing utterly in stemming the onslaught of disease. The strength of a health system is deeply embedded in a nation's political economy. Economic declines or reversals profoundly limit a society's capacity to control disease: GDP per capita moved backward in 54 countries over the decade of the 1990s.[2] Conflict and failed governance devastate the human infrastructure and social trust that enable a health service to function. Beyond politics are many complex reasons for crumbling health systems. Central to the malaise is gross and protracted neglect of the workforce, the key resource driving all health systems.

Fresh opportunities

The crisis of global health, stirring public angst, can provoke political action. With greater public awareness and concern, conditions are being created for faster responses through stronger political commitment, more financial resources, and new mechanisms and actors.

Public concern is pushing for stronger political commitment to health: witness the growing enthusiasm of students in richer countries to work on the health challenges of poorer countries. Medical literacy among key groups, such as people living with HIV/AIDS, has reached levels that enable them to challenge the scientific community and the pharmaceutical industry— with astonishing results. The dramatic fall in prices for antiretroviral drugs reflects in part the effectiveness of social activism and social policy.

Advocacy has pushed global health onto the agenda of high politics. Special sessions of the UN General Assembly and Security Council have

been devoted to HIV/AIDS. The G-8 heads of state have set priorities for global health, including the G-8 Africa Action Plan. Leaders of national governments and regional associations are setting new health goals, such as the 2001 commitment of African leaders in Abuja, Nigeria, to ratchet up their government's health spending.[3]

Embodying the world's commitment to reducing poverty are the Millennium Development Goals (MDGs) endorsed by the UN Millennium Assembly. The goals constitute a global compact among nations of the North and South to achieve eight specific development goals. Health figures prominently among them. Goal 4 targets child mortality, goal 5 maternal health, and goal 6 HIV/AIDS, tuberculosis, malaria, and other diseases.

Political support for the MDGs has been accompanied by a host of new mechanisms— several with tongue-twisting acronyms. Heavily indebted poor country (HIPC) initiatives and poverty reduction strategy papers (PRSPs) fast track donor support and debt reduction to support country-based poverty reduction efforts. National budgets and donor financing are being integrated into medium-term expenditure frameworks (MTEFs) and sector-wide approaches (SWAps), producing general budget support that is consolidating individual projects. Development partners are pledging to promote coordination, mutual accountability, and best practices.

Recent initiatives include the Global Fund to Fight AIDS, Tuberculosis, and Malaria (Global Fund), the Global Alliance on Vaccines and Immunizations (GAVI), and the U.S. President's Emergency Plan for AIDS Relief (PEPFAR). These initiatives are as significant for their new ways of doing business as

❝ For the first time in history, we have the resources and the knowledge to overcome the lethal threats to global health equity

for the enhanced resources they command. The World Bank's Treatment Acceleration Program is also developing new procedures, using civil society to administer antiretroviral treatment in three African countries. The WHO-led 3 by 5 Initiative—to bring 3 million HIV-positive patients under treatment by the end of 2005—is bringing focus and energy to national governments and the entire UN system.

Although few African countries have yet to meet the Abuja target of allocating 15 percent of governmental expenditures to health, many are moving their budgetary allocations in the right direction. Health budgets are moving up. And foreign aid, reversing a long decline, is finally showing its first upswing in a decade.[4] International donors are increasing their spending on health, especially on HIV/AIDS in Africa.

Within five years the Global Fund aims to raise and disburse $7 billion annually. PEPFAR plans to spend $15 billion, about two-thirds of it new money. Debt relief under the HIPC initiative has the potential to increase resource allocations to health, as does unlocking the more than $10 billion in unspent funds languishing in the European Development Fund. An ambitious British-inspired International Finance Facility, if supported by major donors, could provide an additional $50 billion annually for development financing—almost doubling today's aid.

Some of the key obstacles to the poor gaining access to medication are being dismantled. Under sustained pressure from the media and social activists, pharmaceutical companies have brought down the price of antiretroviral drugs. Legal threats against countries that sought to produce or import generic drugs have been dropped. The Doha Declaration on the TRIPS Agreement and Public Health emphasizes that

the agreement on trade-related intellectual property rights should be interpreted so as to protect health and promote access to medicines for all. Although the challenge of drug access continues, the barriers of pricing have come down dramatically, making drugs far more affordable.

Unlike the inability to deal with health threats in previous eras—the Black Death of the 14th century and the influenza epidemic of 1918–19—we have one incalculable advantage today. Our grasp of biomedical sciences and our well-developed public health methods for disease control. For example, in just two decades much has been discovered about the AIDS virus. Simple technologies, such as bed nets against malaria, can be provided more widely than ever. Directly observed treatment, short-course (DOTS) has transformed the prospects for controlling tuberculosis. Antiretroviral treatment is being simplified so that some patients on combination therapy can take just two pills a day.

The information revolution enables decentralized networks to transform our way of doing health work. The internet provides opportunities for remote health stations to tap the medical knowledge bank. Health planning technology is progressing at a fast rate. The old distinction between vertical and horizontal programming is giving way to the recognition that targeting and spending on major health threats, conducted well, can be a means of achieving disease control while building the health infrastructure. Taking antiretroviral treatment to scale is historically unprecedented in public health; lessons can be learned and scaled up speedily. For the first time in history, we have the resources and the knowledge to overcome the lethal threats to global health equity. But will we seize that opportunity?

❝❝ Highly skilled workers are shifting from poorer to richer regions and from the public to the private sector

Health workforce crisis

History will applaud the health workers of the 20th century. It was the commitment, humanity, professionalism, and innovation of several generations of health workers that made possible the dramatic advances in global health. And it is the continuing dedication of millions of health workers, working to prevent diseases, deliver health, and provide a minimum package of services to hundreds of millions of people in poor countries—despite inadequate numbers, poor working conditions, and neglect by policymakers. For many health workers, theirs is not just a job or a career—it is a vocation.

Mirroring today's global health crisis, we face a global crisis of the health workforce. There are not enough health workers, they do not have the right skills and support networks, they are overstretched and overstressed, and often they are not in the right place. What happened? Three major things went wrong: investment was replaced by neglect, the market for health workers went global, and—worst of all—the HIV/AIDS epidemic added horrendous new burdens on precisely those health systems least able to cope.

The triple threat of HIV/AIDS for health care

A genuinely new and uniquely vicious peril to the health workforce has emerged recently: the HIV/AIDS pandemic. This is a three-pronged threat (box 1.1). First, it increases the workload and skill demands on health workers. Hospitals, clinics, and community centers are simply being overwhelmed by AIDS patients. Massive expansion of work in the hardest hit countries is required for new antiretroviral therapy and preventive programs. All available health workers are being mobilized as the ambition and intensity of new HIV/AIDS programs gain support from governments and major donors.

Second, in many countries, health workers are falling ill and dying. Caring for the sick is not only demanding but risky, because of the work-related hazards of contamination. In a few years the HIV prevalence rate among nurses in Lusaka rose from 34 to 44 percent.[5] This hemorrhaging of workers exceeds the current capacity to train new entrants.

Third, health workers have to cope with the psychosocial stress of offering palliative care to increasing numbers of dying patients along with caring for their own sick family and relatives. The immense task of caring for people living with AIDS and rearing children orphaned by AIDS is being absorbed by an army of unremunerated and invisible care-givers—almost all women. In some countries the human fabric of health systems is unraveling.

The acceleration of migration

Health professionals have always been mobile. Leading specialist physicians have long been able to find posts anywhere. What is new is that there is a global market in health workers at many levels, including just-qualified nurses. Like all markets, it is dominated by those with the money to pay. Those who already have health workers are recruiting more, while those who lack workers have even their few health professionals taken away. And this phenomenon is accelerating rapidly.

Highly skilled workers are shifting from poorer to richer regions and from the public to the private sector. The concentration of health professionals in capital cities is well recognized, but regional and international migrations are assuming new dynamics. Anecdotes abound. There are allegedly more Malawian doctors in Manchester than in

❝❝ A shared strategic approach will be required to achieve sustainable solutions for all countries, rich and poor

---

Box 1.1 | **HIV/AIDS: Triple threat to health workers**

"We are here to cure but now with this epidemic we are here to manage it. Even when you discharge a patient, you know he or she will be back. We treat them, and they come back again and are worse off; and we feel powerless because we don't have something to give them."
—*Primary care doctor, South Africa (Ijumba 2003, p. 196)*

The HIV/AIDS epidemic in sub-Saharan Africa is devastating health workers—who face bigger workloads, the loss of colleagues, and the stress of overwork and contamination.

Bigger workloads. HIV/AIDS is generating a huge increase in the disease burden both due to HIV and such related diseases as tuberculosis. In many hospitals across the continent, it is now the greatest source of patients, increasing workloads for all cadres of the health workforce—from medical professionals to laboratory technicians to

counselors to administrative staff. The displacement of many other patients perceived to be less seriously ill has put additional pressures on health centers, with fewer qualified medical personnel. The push to scale up antiretroviral therapy is increasing workloads on top of crumbling systems.

Lost health workers. HIV/AIDS is also depleting the number of health workers in many countries. Death, resignation, and early retirement are the major causes of attrition among health workers. In Malawi 45 percent of health worker deaths were due to AIDS-related illnesses. A recent study suggests that African health systems may lose 20 percent of their workers to HIV/AIDS over the coming few years. In one study, the risk of infection among surgeons was found to be 15 times higher in tropical Africa than in developed countries. Health workers are also leaving their jobs to care for family members and friends or to manage their own illnesses.

Psychosocial stress. The added pressures are a serious risk to health workers with flagging morale and more fatigue, burn-out, and absenteeism. Because few African hospitals have access to antiretroviral drugs, many staff feel that they have gone from healers to death counselors. Fear of being exposed to the disease is discouraging recruitment.

Clearly needed are strategies for reducing staff workloads, creating new cadres of workers, improving incentives and work conditions for existing workers, and training and supporting health workers to cope with the many and ever-changing stresses they face on the job. Most important, however, is to protect health workers from on-the-job exposure to disease—through appropriate training, enforceable safety policies, and adequate supplies of protective gear. Above all, infected workers should have first call on antiretroviral therapy—to save the lives of the lifesavers.

Source: Government of Malawi 2002; Tawfik and Kinoti 2003; Consten and others 1995.

Malawi. And only 50 of 600 Zambian doctors trained since independence continue to practice in the country.[6] Recruitment firms batch together nurses for wholesale export. Doctors in the Philippines are retraining themselves as nurses to pursue lucrative opportunities in changing export markets.[7]

These flows, within and across countries, add to the already severe maldistributions and imbalances. Many low-income countries are losing health staff at an alarming rate. They find themselves relying on only a fraction of the health workers they have trained, whose efforts are now supplemented by foreign nongovernmental organizations (NGOs) and missionaries. Countries well-endowed with health workers are only now considering how to stem these flows or reciprocate. An exceptional case is Cuba, which each year dispatches thousands of medical workers abroad, mostly to African and Caribbean countries.

Although the symptoms are sharpest in poor countries, this is a shared problem. Many wealthy nations depend on imports of workers, and because of the demography of aging in Northern countries, this demand is sure to continue well into the future. In the short term, richer countries are benefiting, but a shared strategic approach will be required to achieve sustainable solutions for all countries, rich and poor.

The relegation to the backwater

For a generation, the people who deliver health have been shockingly neglected. It takes a long time to build up human resources for health, but just a few years to run them down. And in too many places, this is exactly what has happened.

Two decades of health sector "mis-reforms" treated health workers as a cost burden, not an asset. In structural adjustment policies, health reforms imposed ceilings on staff numbers and salaries while capping investment in higher education and training. Human resources became a backwater field for elite policymakers, academics, and scientists—seen as personnel administration, not as science or policy. With the educational pipeline compromised, the health system was further weakened. How could this have happened? Through poor management, inappropriate donor policies, and poor information and knowledge.

Inefficient planning and management of the health workforce, unfortunately, are pervasive problems. And the poor distribution, balance, motivation, skills, and support of health workers are common in countries around the world. In severely affected countries, implementing health interventions at full scale is simply beyond reach, even as drugs and money become more readily available. In sub-Saharan Africa and many low-income countries, the cupboards are now bare. The next phase of health sector reform will have to restock the shelves!

Unhelpful donor and governmental policies are also part of the problem. Many donors consider recurrent spending on human resources only as a fiscal burden, not as an investment, much in the way they looked upon education in the 1970s. The recurring burden bias overlooks the long-term return on most worker-related expenditures. Employing health workers has benefits beyond the immediate services for which they are paid. Their availability, skills, and motivation cannot be turned on and off like tap water.

Although most donor projects use available local talent, they tend to shy away from investing in people for the long term. Instead, they finance technical assistance (often foreign) and short-term training (often fragmented, without strategic vision, coordination, or career planning). In addition, some national governments have their problem practices, including ghost-workers and under-the-table payments for post transfers or medical admissions.

Proper workforce planning demands good data. That too has been neglected, leaving us with great uncertainties surrounding health workers in poor countries.[8] Rapidly changing situations are not well captured by data and evidence, because health is a human process. So the basic tools for

ff **The number, quality, and configuration of human resources shape the output and productivity of health systems**

nurturing a first-class health workforce have rarely been appreciated by policymakers. In all situations, a gender lens is imperative for properly understanding worker motivation, stress, and performance, but too rarely has this been reflected in policy and practice.

We are fortunate in the dedication of so many health workers. Despite worries about physical safety, economic livelihoods, and psychological stress, many frontline workers display enormous dedication and fortitude in the face of hardship. In many cases, they demonstrate leadership and craft innovations under severely constrained circumstances.

Listening to the voices of health workers offers many insights. No one could better represent the experience of being a health care worker—whether in terms of its benefits or its challenges—than health workers themselves. Yet, except among elite physicians, their opinions are rarely sought, their voices often silenced.

Why health workers are so important

Earlier in this chapter we outlined how the international community is recognizing the new challenges of global health, and the new opportunities that have arisen— political leadership, institutions, and money. But so far, international initiatives to tackle the challenges of human resources for health have been conspicuous by their absence. It is a remarkable blind spot.

Outreach services, clinics, and hospitals are only as good as the people who staff them. Health workers are the linchpin, the keystone, the pivot of all efforts to overcome health crises and to achieve the MDGs for health. Only when high-level initiatives, finance, and technologies are matched by an investment in people will the formula for better health for all be credible and effective.

Here we present five major arguments for why health workers matter so much, and then present and analyze data for the impact of health workers on health outcomes.

1. History proves their essential role

The transformation of the workforce into a cluster of science-based, formally organized, well trained, and well compensated professions facilitated the doubling of life expectancy among privileged populations in the last century. In the United States, the *Flexner Report* laid down the scientific foundation of medical practice, and the *Welch-Rose Report* provided a similar basis for public health. Effective disease control programs of the last century were all built on successful human resource strategies (from hookworm to yellow fever, from smallpox to polio). The success of the child survival revolution in the 1980s hinged on mobilizing human resources. In every case of accelerating national health advances, innovative human resource strategies played a role—both in today's high-income countries and in diverse low-income countries, from Costa Rica to China, from Brazil to Iran, and from Chile to India's Kerala state.

2. They spearhead performance

Workers spearhead the performance of health systems, both curative and preventive. The number, quality, and configuration of human resources—informal and community workers, laboratory technicians, and professionals—shape the output and productivity of health systems. Most health workers are committed to social service, and their motivation can be harnessed to achieve better outcomes with limited resources. Often, they serve far beyond the call of duty. They alone have the capacity for communicating with patients and communities—and thus the potential for catalyzing community-driven health transformations. The participation of health workers is especially important in health sector reform. Properly supported, they can be leaders and implement innovation. But treated badly, they can be insurmountable obstacles. When health workers fail, a community can spiral into a health crisis. They must be treated as partners in delivering health, not mere employees.

3. They manage all other health resources
Workers are the ultimate resource in health because they manage and synchronize all other health resources, including financing, technology, information, and infrastructure. It is the health worker who glues these inputs together into a functioning health system (figure 1.2). Neglecting the workforce wastes all other resources. There are already informal reports of vaccines and drugs expiring in warehouses because there are too few workers to deliver the technologies. Of course, workers are not panaceas. They cannot operate effectively without a functioning system of drugs, transport, and support. Complementary inputs have to be synchronized into an operational system for workers to achieve their potential.

But the workforce cannot be considered as simply another input. Health care is a service that is overwhelmingly worker-dependent. As a unique resource, health workers are active agents of health change. They require time and investment to build their capabilities. They are not as responsive to markets as other commodities. And as people they have mixed motivations, which include dedication to service, the desire to contribute

to society, or wanting to advance their own interests. They are not fungible, optional, location-neutral, or immediately available on demand.

4. They command a large share of health budgets
In all health systems, health workers command a significant share of health budgets, in some cases more than 75 percent. In the lowest income countries, staff costs typically exceed two-thirds of the public health budget; the share is likely similar in the private sector. The Dominican Republic's health ministry spends 67 percent of its health budget on health worker salaries, Ecuador's 72 percent.[9] Yet despite their budgetary importance, health workers are often managed as an administrative function through personnel offices focused on procedures. Amazingly, the workforce, commanding the largest share of the budget, is the least strategically planned and managed resource of most health systems. Missing is the recognition that health workers are highly adaptable resources

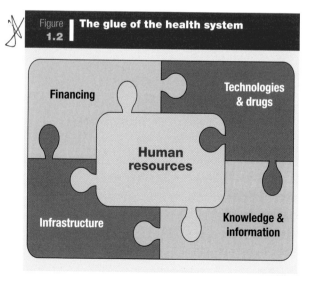

Figure 1.2 | **The glue of the health system**

Financing

Technologies & drugs

Human resources

Infrastructure

Knowledge & information

" Workers report lower burnout, better morale, and greater job satisfaction when the number and quality of staff are adequate

for generating health outputs, reducing waste, and exploiting the huge potential for efficiency gains.

5. They are a main constraint—or contributor—to progress

Health workers are among the principal "binding constraints" for achieving the health-related MDGs. Overcoming the constraint of human resources is necessary but alone insufficient for accelerating progress toward the MDGs. Conversely, strategic management of human resources can be a catalyst for accelerating health progress. Almost all major health breakthroughs in the last century were sparked by the mobilization of health workers.

This chapter also presents some of the accumulating evidence that the density and quality of health workers are major determinants of the health status of populations—that human resources drive health outputs and outcomes, not just anecdotally but in quantitative analysis. Much of this evidence comes from research conducted and reviewed by the JLI.

Empirical data on health workers and health outcomes

Hiring more health workers makes it possible to provide better service. This is no surprise. Of interest and importance are the precise levels at which health worker density makes a difference, and in which ways. These are some of the questions the JLI research set out to answer. Is there a linear relationship between health worker numbers and health outcomes, or a minimum threshold for making a difference? Are particular areas—such as maternal health or infant mortality—especially sensitive to health worker densities? How do

countries compare—can they be fitted into general patterns, and are there over- and under-performers? Can a country be saturated with health professionals—reaching a point at which its people do not demand more workers? And how many health workers are there, who are they, and where are they? JLI research points to answers to many of these crucial questions.

Specific densities of health workers are associated with two key MDG-related health indicators: measles immunization and skilled attendants at birth (figure 1.3). Regression analysis based on worker density and health outputs around the world suggests that a density of about 1.5 workers per 1,000 population is associated with 80 percent coverage with measles immunization, and 2.5 workers per 1,000 with 80 percent coverage of births with skilled attendants. These relationships suggest that a density of 2.5 workers per 1,000 may be considered a threshold of worker density necessary to attain adequate coverage of some essential health interventions and core MDG-related health services.

It can be assumed that more demanding health functions associated with more complex health services—such as antiretroviral therapy—will require higher worker density. This ratio, of course, is only suggestive because the regression does not control for the range of other inputs to health advances—such as socioeconomic progress or new vaccines and drugs. More important, the data omit informal, traditional, and community workers. Nor does the analysis take into account productivity or quality.

Nor do many countries follow the regression precisely. Some perform worse than their worker

❝ A density of 2.5 workers per 1,000 may be considered a threshold of worker density necessary to attain adequate coverage

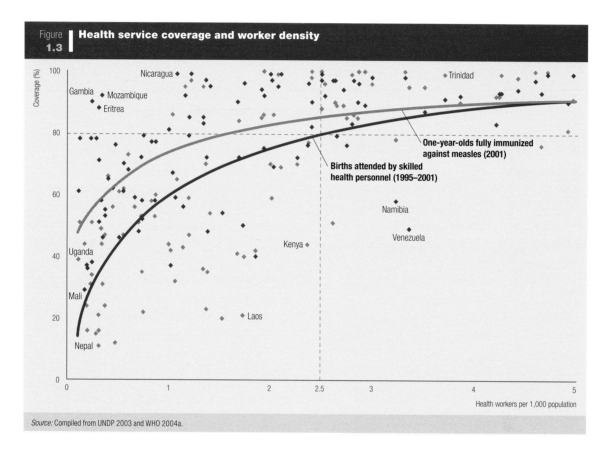

Figure 1.3 | **Health service coverage and worker density**

Coverage (%)

Nicaragua
Gambia ◆ Mozambique
Eritrea
Trinidad

One-year-olds fully immunized against measles (2001)

Births attended by skilled health personnel (1995–2001)

Namibia

Venezuela

Kenya

Uganda

Mali

Laos

Nepal

Health workers per 1,000 population

Source: Compiled from UNDP 2003 and WHO 2004a.

density ratios would suggest. For example, Venezuela and Kenya appear to be under-performing in coverage in comparison to other countries with similar worker densities. Others perform much better. For example, Mozambique, The Gambia, and Eritrea achieve higher coverage than would be predicted by their worker density. Why the deviations? Because of the confounding effects of other social factors, such as education and economics, and of the way countries mobilize and deploy workers not classified under existing international systems. So, the density of 2.5 workers per 1,000 is a suggestive guideline, not a definitive benchmark.

More direct evidence of the importance of worker density and quality for health outcomes comes from studies in hospitals and nursing homes in high-income countries, such as Canada and the United States.[10] Nursing number and quality are measured by hours of nursing care and the education and skill mix of the nursing staff. And health outcomes are measured by length of patient stay, rate of complications, and patient survival to discharge. The findings: higher worker density generates better health outcomes, and workers report lower burnout, better morale, and greater job satisfaction when the number and quality of staff are adequate.

" There does not appear to be any upper cap on consumption of highly skilled and expensive health workers

Figure 1.4 | **Higher income—more health workers**

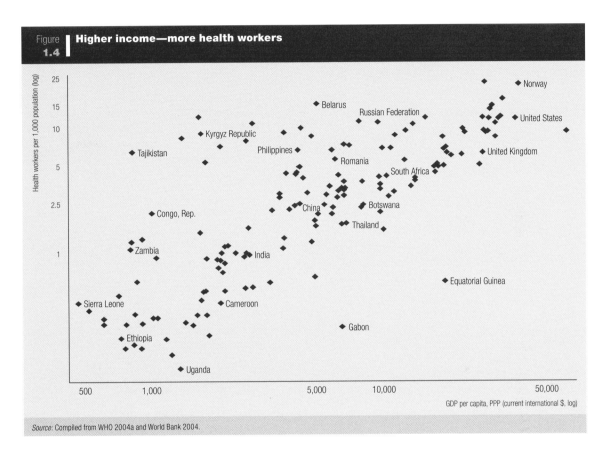

GDP per capita, PPP (current international $, log)

Source: Compiled from WHO 2004a and World Bank 2004.

Studies commissioned by the JLI examined the national patterns of worker density in relation to key variables, such as national income, child and maternal mortality, and expenditure in health care.[11] Not surprisingly, there is a strong relationship between worker density and national income (figure 1.4). Higher income countries have many more doctors, nurses, and midwives per population, just as lower income countries have fewer professional workers. Interestingly, there does not appear to be any upper cap on consumption of highly skilled and expensive health workers. Many of the wealthy high-density countries are major importers of additional workers.

Similarly, the transitional economies of Eastern Europe appear as outliers with higher worker densities than suggested by their national incomes. This may account for some of the shedding of workers now underway in these transitional economies. Most striking are the low-income countries, where low density of workers hinders their capacity to cope with health crisis.

Anand and Baernighausen conducted a quantitative cross-national analysis of human resource density and health status in 118 countries for which data were available (see appendix 2).[12] Lower maternal, infant, and under-five mortality rates are associated with higher income, higher female adult literacy, and lower

“ Health workers are active partners and joint owners in the enterprise of producing good health

income poverty. Controlling for these expected findings, however, the analysis also conclusively showed that human resource density (physicians, nurses, and midwives per 1,000 population) matters significantly in determining these three health outcome measures.

As the density of health workers increases, maternal, infant, and under-five mortality all fall (figure 1.5). The impact of worker density on maternal mortality is the greatest. The analysis suggests that a 10 percent increase in the density of the health workforce is correlated with about a 5 percent decline in maternal mortality. And a 10 percent increase in health worker density is correlated with a 2 percent decline in infant and under-five mortality. Why the stronger effect on maternal mortality? A reasonable hypothesis is that highly trained medical personnel are more essential for the emergency obstetrical services to avert maternal deaths than for the simpler tasks, such as immunizations for infant and child health.

Workers as a global health trust

Health workers help people produce their own health by linking them to information, to vaccines and drugs, and to caring and humane services. Performing these critical functions the world over, they can be viewed as a "global health trust." The term "trust" underscores the fact that workers are the essential human asset base for the production of good health. Also, human trust and empathy lie at the heart of the relationship between a health worker and the person served.

Unlike funds, medicines, or infrastructure, health workers are active partners and joint owners in the enterprise of producing good health. Their input is qualitatively different and quantitatively critical. To be effective, they must be well distributed, motivated, skilled, and supported.

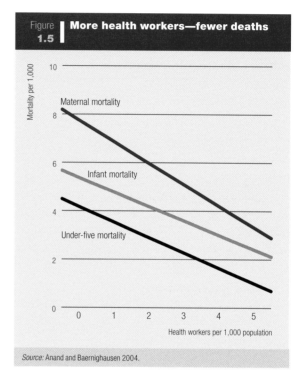

Figure 1.5 | **More health workers—fewer deaths**

Source: Anand and Baernighausen 2004.

For the JLI, the importance of human resources in health is axiomatic. Our challenge is to substantiate the case for making health workers a priority. This requires answering some questions. Who are the world's health workers? How many are they, with what skills, and where? What patterns are there in national health workforces? And what are the measurable outcomes of different densities and patterns of health workers? We found remarkably little evidence on all these questions. But there was enough to map the outlines of the situation today and the challenges we face.

Who are the health workers?

Our first challenge was to define health workers. This proved far more complicated than anticipated, as there is no standard definition for who is a health

❝ We estimate the global health workforce at more than 100 million workers; the world had 9 million doctors and 15 million nurses and midwives in 2000

worker. Indeed, we estimate that for every formally qualified doctor or nurse, there are at least three or more uncounted health workers, including the "invisible" health workers at family level, informal and traditional healers, and a range of community health workers without professional qualification. Any policy measures aiming to improve the health workforce and enhance health outcomes must take this fundamental fact into account.

The challenge of identifying who actually delivers health proved sufficiently important and complex that an entire chapter of this report (chapter 2, "Communities at the Frontlines") is devoted to its exploration.

How many health workers?

The world's stock of all health workers at any given time represents the summation of many moving parts comprising inflows and outflows. Currently available workers display various attributes: geographic and public-private distribution, and balances in skill mix, gender composition, and work teams. These attributes—with the strategic planning and management that give workers incentives in a supportive work environment—determine the efficient, effective, and equitable generation of good health services.

This overall stock of workers is regulated by inflows and outflows at both national and global levels (figure 1.6). Inflows are determined by the pace of graduates produced by educational institutions and pre-service training programs or added through in-migration. Outflows are due to retirement, death, or out-migration. These flows have powerful time dynamics. Outflows or attrition can be very rapid—for example, through premature deaths due to AIDS or through mass out-migration.

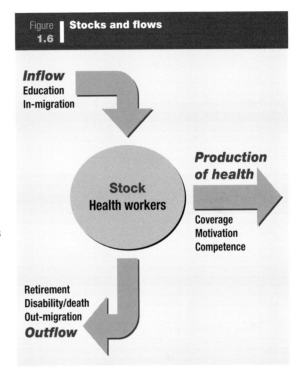

Figure 1.6 | Stocks and flows

Inflow
Education
In-migration

Stock
Health workers

Production of health

Coverage
Motivation
Competence

Retirement
Disability/death
Out-migration
Outflow

Inflows or intakes can be time-consuming, expensive, and dependent on strong educational institutions. Only importing professionals can build up worker numbers without significant time delays or monetary investments—filling the pipeline for producing professionals can require a decade or more. These dynamics explain why HIV/AIDS, global mobility, and chronic underinvestment are decimating the workforce in some of the world's poorest countries.

Applying these definitions and metrics, we estimate the global health workforce at more than 100 million workers. Added to the 24 million enumerated doctors, nurses, and midwives are at least 75 million more uncounted informal, traditional, community, and allied workers. According to statistics compiled by the WHO, the world had 9 million doctors and 15

❝ Many countries in sub-Saharan Africa have the same number or fewer health workers today than they did 30 or even 40 years ago

million nurses and midwives in 2000.[13] These counts give an average world density of 1.6 doctors and 2.5 nurses per 1,000 population. The ratio of nurses to doctors is 1.6 to 1.0. With the last published global survey estimating 2.3 million doctors in 1971, the 2000 data suggest that the global pool of doctors has been growing on average at about 5 percent a year.[14]

Unfortunately, many health workers—some say the more important ones—are not counted in official statistics. Omitted are community health workers, medical and nursing auxiliaries, informal workers, traditional practitioners, and nonmedical staff—in other words, entire cadres of informal and community workers. Because these workers are excluded from the statistics, caution should be exercised in interpreting global data on the workforce.

Appendix 2 describes the WHO's suggested guidelines, which are not uniformly applied across diverse countries. For example, nurses and midwives are sometimes categorized separately, sometimes together. For this analysis, therefore, all nursing and midwifery counts are combined and listed as "nursing." The measure that seems to offer some robustness is to combine the total counts of all doctors, nurses, and midwives. This approximate measure of worker numbers and density is used throughout this report.

Where are the world's health workers?

If a global minister of health were to survey the world and allocate the 100 million health workers across the world according to health needs, she would not come up with the distribution that exists today. The geographical locations and skill mixes reflect past histories of public policy and training,

today's global marketplace for labor, and a range of political and economic factors. The global maldistribution of workers reflects inequities even more marked than inequities in health status.

Whatever count is most valid, the severe maldistribution of health workers is obvious. Asia, with about 50 percent of the world's people, has 30 percent of the global stock of doctors, nurses, and midwives. Together, Europe and North America have 20 percent of the world's people, but almost half of the physicians and 60 percent of the nurses. For doctors and nurses the regional differences are enormous. Average density is 1 worker per 1,000 population in sub-Saharan Africa, but more than 10 per 1,000 in Europe and North America (figure 1.7). Country densities vary even more. Doctors range from a high of 6 per 1,000 in Italy to a low of 0.02 per 1,000 in Rwanda. Nurse and midwife density ranges from 22 per 1,000 population in Finland to a representative low of only 0.09 nurses and midwives per 1,000 in Uganda—a more than 200-fold difference. The atlas of countries colored according to worker density vividly underscores these global inequalities (figure 1.8).

Of equal concern: some world regions are losing ground over time. Many countries in sub-Saharan Africa have the same number or fewer health workers today than they did 30 or even 40 years ago. In many countries, this declining stock of workers is coupled with the additional health needs of the population amid disease, famine, and conflict-related crises.[15] Other developing country regions seemed to have fared better. Although fewer than 10 percent of doctors were in the "developing world" in 1971, most countries in Asia,

" Often magnifying the geographic imbalances are within-country workforce inequalities in gender, ethnicity, skill mix, and private and public sector employment

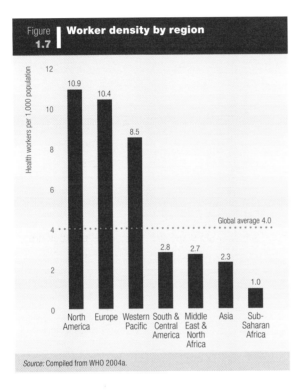

Figure 1.7 | Worker density by region

Health workers per 1,000 population

North America 10.9
Europe 10.4
Western Pacific 8.5
South & Central America 2.8
Middle East & North Africa 2.7
Asia 2.3
Sub-Saharan Africa 1.0

Global average 4.0

Source: Compiled from WHO 2004a.

in government positions. Since there are almost no doctors or nurses in the private sector outside urban centers, the overall urban concentration of providers is even greater than for the public sector alone.[19] In Mexico an estimated 15 percent of all physicians are unemployed, underemployed, or inactive—yet rural posts remain unfilled.[20]

Often magnifying the geographic imbalances are within-country workforce inequalities in gender, ethnicity, skill mix, and private and public sector employment. While some countries have one doctor for five nurses, as in Thailand and South Africa, other countries may have three doctors for each nurse. Important for team and task delegations, the skill mix profoundly influences a health system's efficiency. Still other countries suffer from negative work environments that make maldistributions worse and reduce productivity. In nearly all situations, the information and data are extremely limited, handicapping understanding and country-based policy, planning, and programs.

Five clusters of countries

The JLI research mapped countries according to health worker density and health outcomes. Depending on a host of factors, there is extreme variability. The patterns we find indicate five major clusters of similar countries. At the extremes we see countries with many health workers and high life expectancies (such as the most developed nations), and countries with few health workers and poor health (such as the poorest nations in sub-Saharan Africa). But in between, there are many variations and a few surprises.

These comparisons and clusters can help in seeking common lessons, easily shared

Latin America, and the Middle East have seen their relative position improve in recent decades.[16]

Adding to the global disparities are intranational inequalities in the distribution of the health workforce. Access to health care in rural, remote, and marginal locations is constrained by worker and facility allocation patterns which commonly favor urban centers. In Nicaragua, for instance, 50 percent of the country's health personnel are in the capital city of Managua, home to only 20 percent of the people.[17] In Ghana, more than 85 percent of general physicians work in urban regions, although 66 percent of the population lives in rural areas.[18] In Bangladesh, metropolitan centers have around 15 percent of the country's population, but 35 percent of doctors and 30 percent of nurses

1

Figure
1.8 | **Human resources and health clusters**

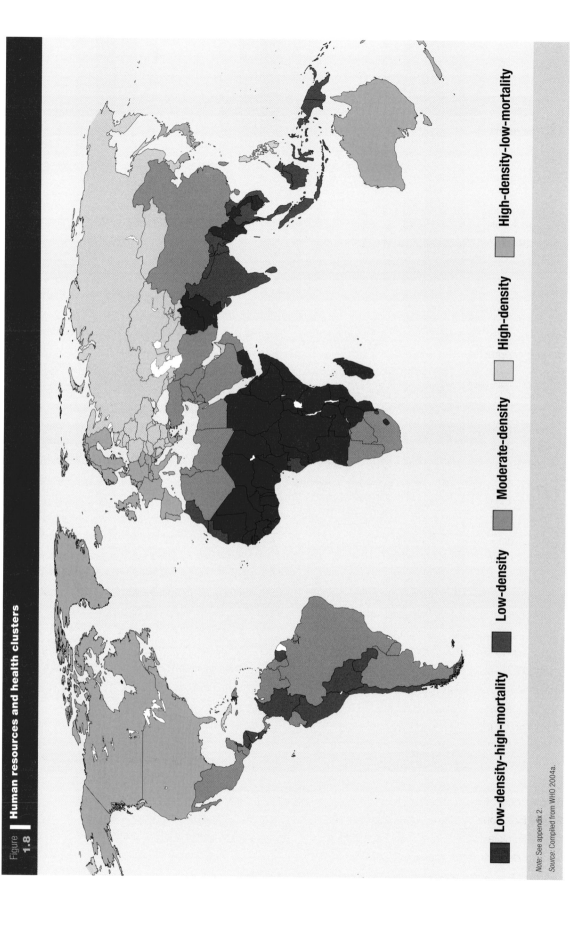

Low-density-high-mortality   **Low-density**   **Moderate-density**   **High-density**   **High-density-low-mortality**

Note: See appendix 2.
Source. Compiled from WHO 2004a.

❝ There are no clear 'developed' versus 'developing' country patterns—indeed, the global pattern suggests a continuum along worker density and mortality

across national boundaries to shape solutions to local circumstances. Understanding such national patterns in the global context is a critical strategic factor in designing national strategies. One size clearly does not fit all!

Different criteria can be used to cluster countries according to their human resource endowments, such as geography (world continents) and income (GDP) or economic, political, and cultural dimensions.[21] Because this report focuses on health workers, we developed country clusters based on human resources and health status. Figure 1.9 depicts the clustering criteria employed with arbitrarily selected cutoff levels of 2.5 and 5.0 workers per 1,000. The lower boundary approximates the minimal density associated with 80 percent coverage of key health services linked to immunization and maternal health. The upper boundary exceeds the global average density of 4 workers per 1,000. Among the low and high density groups, those with either high or low under-five mortality levels are also separated. Using these cutoffs, our analysis generated five basic clusters for 186 countries: low-density-high-mortality, low-density, moderate-density, high-density, and high-density-low-mortality.

Each of these five clusters is described below (a detailed list of countries is in appendix 2).

Low density and high mortality. Of the 45 countries in this cluster, 37 are in sub-Saharan Africa, including the Democratic Republic of Congo, Mozambique, and Sierra Leone. The non-African countries in this cluster include wartorn Afghanistan and politically unstable Haiti.

Low density. Most of these 30 countries are in Asia (India, Bangladesh, and Vietnam) and

the Americas (Bolivia, Chile, and Paraguay), although a few are in sub-Saharan Africa.

Moderate density. The 42 countries in this cluster are found largely in Central and South America and the Eastern Mediterranean. They include Brazil, Jamaica, Mexico, and Turkey.

High density. A majority of these 35 countries are former Soviet transitional economies shifting from socialist to mixed private-public systems, such as Lithuania and Ukraine. In this cluster are two socialist countries, Cuba and the Democratic People's Republic of Korea, and exporting countries such as Cuba and the Philippines. Cuba falls very close to the high-density-low-mortality cluster.

High density and low mortality. Largely in Western Europe and North America, the 34 countries in this cluster are mostly members of the OECD, including Canada, Spain, and Japan.

Noteworthy is the fact that there are no clear "developed" versus "developing" country patterns. Indeed, the global pattern suggests a continuum along worker density and mortality. Within developing countries are 30-fold or greater differences in worker density. The density of doctors in Chile and Peru, for example, approaches that of the United Kingdom and is almost twice that of nearby Bolivia. And unlike regions of Africa or Asia, their nursing density is quite low, a consistent pattern throughout Latin American countries.

Clearly, workforce planning and management must be finetuned to the unique circumstances of diverse countries. Of primary concern are countries struggling with the double crisis of growing health threats and rising mortality with feeble health systems unable to respond to deteriorating conditions.

> **All countries, rich as well as poor, suffer from numeric, skill, and geographic imbalances of their workforces**

1

Figure
1.9 | **Five clusters**

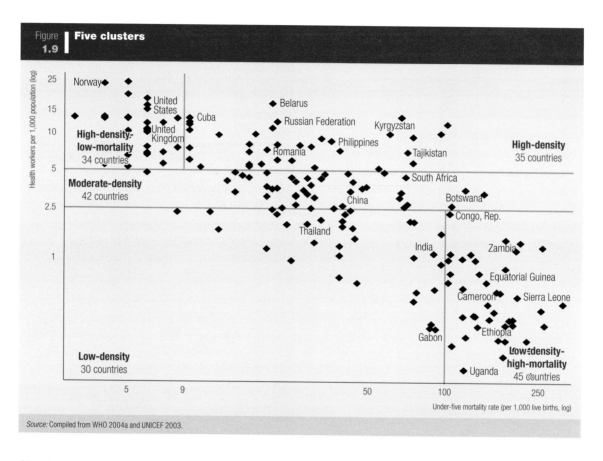

Source: Compiled from WHO 2004a and UNICEF 2003.

Challenges

The JLI research findings do not paint a complete picture. There is too little evidence, and our brushstrokes are too broad for the kind of detail that is necessary for a national health planner. But the outlines of the landscape are becoming clear. We can begin to answer some fundamental questions.

Should there be global norms and standards of numeric adequacy of workers? Can we define what would be considered a worker surplus or worker shortage? Our answer begins with a cautionary "no," and then a specification of how and why we can say "yes."

Start with the cautionary "no." To make these judgments would require global norms or standards, defined by health needs or market demand for workers. We conclude that country diversity argues against a single global norm or standard (box 1.2). Instead, a range of worker numbers and compositions is feasible for countries with diverse health challenges and diverse legacies of health workers and health systems.

Rather than a single norm or standard, there appears to be a range of adequate or optimal densities for diverse countries to maintain well functioning health systems. Rather than an optimum

❝ **We estimate the global shortage at more than 4 million workers; sub-Saharan African countries must nearly triple their current numbers of workers by urgently adding at least 1 million workers**

mix, one could argue for a "minimum threshold" of worker density as essential for the provision of core health services related to achieving the MDGs. For example, one could postulate that to achieve 80 percent coverage of the population with skilled attendants at birth, a minimum threshold of 2.5 workers per 1,000 population would be required. For illustrative purposes, we have adopted this arbitrary baseline to underscore the magnitude of health workers deficiencies in hard-pressed countries around the world.

All countries, rich as well as poor, suffer from numeric, skill, and geographic imbalances of their workforces. All countries can accelerate health gains by more strategically investing in and managing their health workforce. In this report, we adopt a global perspective while focusing on low-density-high-mortality countries with severe worker shortages because of the urgency of their dire health situations.

Now we can give our qualified "yes" and specify the true global challenges, the fields in which international targets can meaningfully be set.

We conclude that our most outstanding challenges are to address five problems:

- *There is a massive global shortage of workers.* While the data limit quantitative precision, we estimate the global shortage at more than 4 million workers. Sub-Saharan African countries must nearly triple their current numbers of workers by urgently adding the equivalent of at least 1 million workers if they are to begin to even approach achieving the MDGs for health (box 1.3).
- *Nearly all countries suffer from skill imbalances, creating huge inefficiencies.* In some countries the skill mix depends

---

| Box 1.2 | **Norms or standards?** |

There is no agreement among international organizations of any single norm or standard for worker numbers that determine surplus or shortages. Nor are there norms or standards for patterns or teams of workers for various national epidemiologic patterns. In *World Development Report 1993: Investing in Health* (p. 139) the World Bank recommended that "public health and minimum essential clinical interventions require about 0.1 physician per 1,000 population and between 2 and 4 graduate nurses per physician." But there does not appear to be any empirical evidence to substantiate this recommendation.

In the United States it has been recommended that one primary care doctor be available for each 3,500 population to be served; counties with fewer doctors are considered to have a personnel shortage (American Academy of Family Physicians 2000). Experience around the world demonstrates that worker density relates to many factors beyond equity and efficiency in health system performance. For example, "health maintenance organizations in the United States operate with 1.2 physicians per 1,000 enrollees, compared with 4.5 physicians in the fee-for-service sector" (World Bank 1993, p. 139).

---

excessively on doctors and specialists. In most countries population-based public health workers are neglected. Many countries should revamp their health systems toward a workforce that more closely reflects the health needs of their populations by deploying auxiliary and community workers.

- *Nearly all countries suffer from maldistribution made worse by unplanned migration.* Urban concentrations are a problem for all countries. Improving within-country equity requires

❝ **The lack of information hampers planning, policies, and programs—this deficiency must be remedied**

| Box 1.3 | **"Shortages"— giving a sense of scale** |

What constitutes a "shortage?" And how can it be quantified? The concept of shortage depends on what is considered adequate. Moreover, shortage is a relative term influenced by other variables such as imbalances, maldistribution, and worker performance. This report quantifies shortages—globally and regionally—not to seek numeric precision but to offer a sense of the scale of gaps.

We use an arbitrary minimum worker density threshold of 2.5 workers (doctors, nurses, and midwives) per 1,000 population. Computations based on this threshold provides a numeric sense of the scale of the challenges. Caution is indicated not to misinterpret the estimated "shortage." Other levels could have been selected; the WHO data base counts only professional categories, with many workers uncounted. Nor do numeric counts say anything about unproductive workers or unfilled vacancies even though many trained workers may be unemployed in a country. Critically important in considering shortages are strategies to improve worker retention, productivity,

and the work environment. Without such improvements, attaining numeric worker targets will fail like pouring water into a leaking bucket.

Accepting these caveats, we estimate a world shortage of about 4 million health workers. This number would bring 75 countries containing 2.5 billion people to a minimum threshold of 2.5 workers per 1,000 population; sub-Saharan Africa would require the equivalent of 1 million additional workers. Sub-Saharan Africa currently has roughly 600,000 physicians, nurses, and midwives, which translates to a worker density of about 1.0 per 1,000 population. While home to about 10 percent of the world's people, the region has only 1 percent of the world's physicians and 3 percent of the world's nurses and midwives. This estimation of Africa's numeric deficiency is similar in magnitude to another research study using different methods that called for at least 1.4 million additional physicians and nurses required to meet the MDG's target reduction in infant mortality (Kurowski 2004).

An important conclusion of the numeric approach is the stark

realization that national strategies that focus on doctors and nurses are not feasible for most low-density-high-mortality countries. Simple computations of production rates of doctors, nurses, and midwives in sub-Saharan Africa demonstrate the Herculean challenge of accelerating educational efforts to achieve this minimum threshold. Tanzania, which has a relatively high density of workers among African countries, faces a shortfall of 35,000 workers to reach the threshold. To fill this gap by 2015—with no attrition from the current workforce—would take an average annual production of 3,500 physicians, nurses, and midwives. Current levels of production in the country are less than one-fifth this number, with about 90 physicians and 550 nurses and midwives graduating each year.

Innovative approaches will have to be developed with a fundamental realignment of the health workforce. Africa's future—by necessity and practicality—must be based on auxiliary cadres such as community health workers—appropriately motivated, distributed, and skilled.

Source: Compiled by the Joint Learning Initiative from WHO 2004a, Kurowski 2004, and Wyss 2004a.

attracting health workers to rural and marginal communities. In some countries, there is also maldistribution between public and private sectors. International equity is severely challenged by unplanned

international migration—as the depletion of nurses and doctors cripples health systems in poorer sending countries.

- *Nearly all countries are handicapped by negative work environments.* They must scale

❝❝ Strategic planning and management of human resources at all levels can generate huge efficiency gains for health

up good practices to strengthen professional incentives, work incentives, and financial and nonfinancial incentives. Workers must be provided with drugs, equipment, and supplies. Their voices must be heard.

- *The weak knowledge base vitiates possibilities for greater effectiveness.* Information on workers is sparse, data fragmentary, research limited. The lack of information hampers planning, policies, and programs—this deficiency must be remedied.

In the three chapters that follow, this report focuses on these challenges. The chapters examine, in sequence, communities at the frontlines, country leadership, and global responsibilities. Beginning with the health of an individual and family, each successive aggregation—community, nation, and globe—offers additional opportunities and broadens shared responsibilities. The final chapter proposes an agenda for action to harness the power of health workers for equitable health and development.

Throughout the report, we underscore that strategic planning and management of human resources at all levels can generate huge efficiency gains for health. Evidence shows, for example, a three-fold difference in health outcomes such as under-five mortality rates among countries with very similar total health expenditures within the low-density-high-mortality cluster. Similarly, many different levels of mortality and health expenditures are possible among countries with similar worker densities. These efficiency gains appear most feasible within country cluster groupings. In other words, poorer countries need not attempt to attain the numeric density of wealthier countries in order to achieve better health outcomes. Strengthening the

competencies, coverage, and motivation of existing and rapidly mobilized health workers can generate significant health gains.

While global in perspective, this report focuses on communities and countries in health crisis—mostly sub-Saharan African countries in the low-density-high-mortality cluster. These countries have high disease burden, rising mortality, severe worker shortages and imbalances, weak educational and financial institutions, and high dependence on donors and external forces. The indivisibility and solidarity of global health depend on how we as a world community respond to these challenges.

Notes

1. de Waal and Whiteside 2003.
2. UNDP 2003.
3. NEPAD 2001.
4. Michaud 2003.
5. Ndongko and Oladepo 2003.
6. WHO 2004c.
7. Chan 2003.
8. Narasimhan and others 2004.
9. Berman and others 1999.
10. Blegen and others 1998; Harrington and others 2000; Aiken and others 2002a; Aiken and others 2002b; Needleman 2002; Cho and others 2003; McGillis Hall and others 2003; Sasichay-Akkadechanunt and others 2003.
11. JLI 2004.
12. Anand and Baernighausen 2004.
13. WHO 2004a.
14. Mejia and Pizurki 1976.
15. Liese and Dussault 2004.
16. Mejia and Pizurki 1976.
17. Nigenda and Machado 2000.
18. WHO 1997.
19. Bangladesh Ministry of Health and Family Welfare 1997.
20. WHO 2000.
21. Roemer 1991.

References

Aiken, Linda H., Sean P. Clarke, and Douglas M. Sloane. 2002a. "Hospital Staffing, Organization, and Quality of Care: Cross-National Findings." *International Journal for Quality in Health Care* 14 (1): 5–13.

Aiken, Linda H., Sean P. Clarke, Douglas M. Sloane, Julie Sochalski, and Jeffrey H. Silber. 2002b. "Hospital Nurse Staffing and Patient Mortality, Nurse Burnout, and Job Dissatisfaction." *Journal of the American Medical Association* 288 (16): 1987–93.

American Academy of Family Physicians. 2000. *The United States Relies on Family Physicians, Unlike any Other Specialty.* Policy Center One-Pager, no. 5. The Robert Graham Center, Policy Studies in Family Medicine and Primary Care, Washington, D.C.

Anand, Sudhir, and Till Baernighausen. 2004. "Human Resources and Health Outcomes: Cross-Country Econometric Study." *The Lancet* 364 (9445): 1603–9.

Bangladesh, Ministry of Health and Family Welfare. 1997. *Human Resources Development in Health and Family Planning in Bangladesh: A Strategy for Change.* Human Resources Development Unit, Dhaka.

Beaglehole, Robert, and Mario R. Dal Poz. 2003. "Public Health Workforce: Challenges and Policy Issues." *Human Resources for Health* 1 (1): 4.

Berman, Peter, Lisa Arellanes, Pamela Henderson, and Alessandro Magnoli. 1999. *Health Care Financing in Eight Latin American and Caribbean Nations: The First Regional National Health Accounts Network.* LAC/HSR Health Sector Reform Initiative. [www.lachealthaccounts.org/files/480_16hsrpres8studies.pdf].

Blegen, Mary A., Colleen J. Goode, and Laura Reed. 1998. "Nurse Staffing and Patient Outcomes." *Nursing Research* 47 (1): 43–50.

Campos, Francisco. "Utilization and Effectiveness of the Spectrum of Health Workers." Universidade Federal de Minas Gerais Núcleo de Pesquisa em Saúde Coletiva, Brazil. Joint Learning Initiative Working Paper. [www.globalhealthtrust.org].

Chan, Danny. 2003. "Philippine Doctors Study Nursing to Land U.S. Jobs." SikhSpectrum.com Issue 10. [www.sikhspectrum.com/]

Cho, S. H., S. Ketefian, V. H. Barkauskas, and D. G. Smith. 2003. "The Effects of Nurse Staffing on Adverse Events, Morbidity, Mortality, and Medical Costs." *Nursing Research* 52 (2): 71–79.

Commission on Macroeconomics and Health. 2001. *Macroeconomics and Health: Investing in Health for Economic Development.* Geneva: World Health Organization.

Consten, E. C., J. J. van Lanschot, P. C. Henny, J. G. Tinnemans, and J. T. van der Meer. 1995. "A Prospective Study on the Risk of Exposure to HIV during Surgery in Zambia." *AIDS* 9 (6): 585–8.

de Waal, Alex, and Alan Whiteside. 2003. "New Variant Famine: AIDS and Food Crisis in Southern Africa." *The Lancet* 362 (9391): 1234–37.

Diallo, Khassoum, Pascal Zurn, Neeru Gupta, and Mario Dal Poz. 2003. "Monitoring and Evaluation of Human Resources for Health: An International Perspective." *Human Resources for Health* 1 (1): 3.

Dussault, Gilles, and Carl-Ardy Dubois. 2003. "Human Resources for Health Policies: A Critical Component in Health Policies." *Human Resources for Health* 1 (1): 1.

Dussault, Gilles, and Félix Rigoli. 2002. "Dimensiones laborales de las reformas sectoriales en salud: sus relaciones con eficiencia, equidad y calidad." *Revista Latinoamericana de Estudios del Trabajo, El mundo del trabajo en el ámbito de la salud* 8 (15): 15–45.

Egger, Dominique, and Orvill Adams. 1999. "Imbalances in Human Resources for Health: Can Policy Formulation and Planning Make a Difference?" *Human Resources for Health Development Journal* 3 (1): 52–68.

Flexner, Abraham. 1910. *Medical Education in the United States and Canada.* Boston: Merrymount Press.

Gupta, Neeru, Khassoum Diallo, Pascal Zurn, and Mario R. Dal Poz. 2003. "Assessing Human Resources for Health: What Can Be Learned from Labour Force Surveys?" *Human Resources for Health* 1 (1): 5.

Haines, Andy, and Andrew Cassels. 2004. "Can the Millennium Development Goals Be Attained?" *British Medical Journal* 329 (7462): 394–7.

Harrington, Charlene, David Zimmerman, Sarita L. Karon, James Robinson, and Patricia Beutel. 2000. "Nurse Home Staffing and Its Relationship to Deficiencies." *Journal of Geronotology* 55B(5): S278-S287.

Hossain, Belayet, and Khaleda Begum. 1998. "Survey of the Existing Health Workforce of Ministry of Health, Bangladesh." *Human Resources Development Journal* 2 (2): 109–16.

Ijumba, Petrida. 2003. "'Voices of Primary Health Care Facility Workers." In P. Ijumbe, A. Ntuli, and P. Barron, eds., *South African Health Review 2002.* Durban: Health Systems Trust. [www.hst.org.za/sahr].

Joint Learning Initiative. 2004. JLI Commissioned Papers available at [www.globalhealthtrust.org].

Kurowski, Christoph. 2004. *Scope, Characteristics and Policy Implications of the Health Worker Shortage in Low-Income Countries of Sub-Saharan Africa.* Joint Learning Initiative Working Paper. World Bank, Washington, D.C. [www.globalhealthtrust.org].

Liese, Bernhard, and Gilles Dussault. 2004. "The State of the Health Workforce in Sub-Saharan Africa: Evidence of Crisis and Analysis of Contributing Factors." Africa Region Human Development Working Paper 75. World Bank, Washington, D.C.

Malawi, Government of. 2002. "Impact of HIV/AIDS on Human Resources in the Malawi Public Sector." Malawi Government and United Nations Development Programme. New York.

McGillis Hall, L., D. Doran, R. G. Baker, G. H. Pink, S. Sidani, L. O'Brien-Pallas, and G. J. Donner. 2003. "Nurse Staffing Models as Predictors of Patient Outcomes." *Medical Care* 41 (9): 1096–1109.

McNeil, Jr., Donald G. 2002. "Global War on AIDS Runs Short of Key Weapon." *New York Times*. October 9.

Mejia, A., and H. Pizurki. 1976. *World Migration of Health Manpower.* World Health Organization Chronicle 30:455–60.

Michaud, Catherine. 2003. "Development Assistance for Health: Recent Trends and Resource Allocation." World Health Organization, Geneva.

MSF (Médecins Sans Frontières). 2002. "From Durban to Barcelona: Overcoming the Treatment Deficit." Policy Document, 14th International HIV/AIDS Conference 2002, Barcelona. July 2002.

Narasimhan, Vasant, Hilary Brown, Ariel Pablos-Mendez, Orvill Adams, Gilles Dussault, Gijs Elzinga, Anders Nordstrom, Demissie Habte, Marian Jacobs, Giorgio Solimano, Nelson Sewankambo, Suwit Wibulpolprasert, Timothy Evans, and Lincoln Chen. 2004. "Responding to the Global Human Resources Crisis." *The Lancet* 363 (9419): 1469–72.

Ndongko, W., and O. Oladepo. 2003. "Impact of HIV/AIDS on Public Sector Capacity in Sub-Saharan Africa: Towards a Framework for the Protection of Public Sector Capacity and Effective Response to the Most Affected Countries." Africa Capacity Building Foundation, Board of Governors. 13th Annual Meeting, June 29, 2004, The Hague.

Needleman, Jack, Peter Buerhaus, Soeren Mattke, Maureen Stewart, and Katya Zelevinsky. 2002. "Nurse-Staffing Levels and the Quality of Care in Hospitals." *New England Journal of Medicine* 346 (22): 1715–22.

NEPAD (New Partnership for Africa's Development). 2001. "The New Partnership for Africa's Development (NEPAD)." Abuja, October 21. [www.au2002.gov.za/docs/key_oau/nepad.pdf].

Nigenda, G., and H. Machado. 2000. "From State to Market: The Nicaraguan Labour Market for Health Personnel." *Health Policy and Planning* 15 (3): 312–18.

Rockefeller Foundation. 1915. *Welch-Rose Report on Schools of Public Health.* New York.

Roemer, Milton I. 1991. *National Health Systems of the World: Volume I: The Countries.* Oxford: Oxford University Press.

———. 1993. *National Health Systems of the World: Volume II: The Issues.* Oxford: Oxford University Press.

Sasichay-Akkadechanunt, T., C. C. Scalzi, and A. F. Jawad. 2003. "The Relationship Between Nursing Staffing and Patient Outcomes." *Journal of Nursing Administration* 33 (9): 478–85.

Shisana, O., and L. Simbayi. 2002. *South African National HIV Prevalence, Behavioural Risks and Mass Media— Household Survey 2002.* Research report. Cape Town: South African Human Sciences Research Council.

Shisana, O., E. Hall, K. R. Maluleke, D. J. Stoker, C. Schwabe, M. Colvin, J. Chauveau, C. Botha, T. Gumede, H. Fomundam, N. Shaikh, T. Rehle, E. Udjo, and D. Grisselquist. 2003. *The Impact of HIV/AIDS on the Health Sector: National Survey of Health Personnel, Ambulatory and Hospitalised Patients and Health Facilities 2002.* Pretoria: National Department of Health.

Tawfik, Linda, and Stephen N. Kinoti. 2003. "The Impact of HIV/AIDS on the Health Workforce in Sub-Saharan Africa: Support for Analysis and Research in Africa Project (SARA)." U.S. Agency for International Development, Washington, D.C.

UNDP (United Nations Development Programme). 1994. *Human Development Report 1994: New Dimensions of Human Security.* New York: Oxford University Press.

———. 2003. *Human Development Report 2003: Millennium Development Goals: A Compact Among Nations to End Human Poverty.* New York: Oxford University Press.

UNICEF (United Nations Children's Fund). 2003. *State of the World's Children 2003.* New York.

USAID (U.S. Agency for International Development). 1999. Accelerating the Implementation of HIV/AIDS Prevention and Mitigation Programs in Africa. Draft Working Paper. USAID Bureau for Africa and USAID Global Bureau, Washington, D.C.

———. 2003. "The Health Sector Human Resources Crisis in Africa: An Issues Paper." USAID Bureau of Africa, Office of Sustainable Development.

Van Lerberghe, Wim, Orvill Adams, and Paulo Ferrinho. 2002. "Human Resources Impact Assessment."

Bulletin of the World Health Organization 80 (7): 525.

WHO (World Health Organization). 1997. *Inter-Country Consultation on Development of Human Resources in Health in the Africa Region.* Accra.

———. 2000. *World Health Report 2000: Health Systems: Improving Performance.* Geneva.

———. 2003a. *World Health Report 2003: Shaping the Future.* Geneva.

———. 2003b. "Key Aspects on the Classification of Human Resources for Health." Draft. Human Resources for Health/OSD/EIP, WHO/HQ, Geneva.

———. 2004a. "WHO Estimates of Health Personnel: Physicians, Nurses, Midwives, Dentists, Pharmacists." WHO Headquarters, Geneva. [www.who.int/globalatlas/autologin/hrh_login.asp].

———. 2004b. "Gender and the Global Health Workforce: Information from 3 Key Sources." Geneva.

———. 2004c. "Human Resources for Health Country Synthesis Report." Draft. Paper prepared for the High Level Forum Meeting for Health MDGs. Geneva.

World Bank. 1993. *World Development Report 1993: Investing in Health.* New York: Oxford University Press.

———. 2004. *World Development Indicators 2004.* Washington, D.C.

Wyss, Kaspar. 2004a. "Human Resources for Health Development for Scaling-up Anti-Retroviral Treatment in Tanzania." Report for the Department Human Resources for Health of the World Health Organization, Geneva.

———. 2004b. "An Approach to Classifying Human Resources Constraints to Attaining Health-Related Millennium Development Goals." *Human Resources for Health* 2 (11): 6.

Zurn, Pascal, Mario Dal Poz, Barbara Stilwell, and Orvill Adams. 2002. "Imbalances in the Health Workforce: Briefing Paper." World Health Organization, Geneva. [www.who.int/hrh/documents/en/imbalances_briefing.pdf].

Communities
at the frontlines

Since ancient times in all civilizations, some members of the community have been singled out to assist people through the passages of life

CHAPTER two

Communities at the Frontlines

Since ancient times in all civilizations, some members of the community have been singled out to assist people through the passages of life—birth, illness, and death—sharing in moments of joy and satisfaction, suffering and pain, sickness and recovery. The knowledge and skills for managing these passages have been passed down through oral tradition and popular culture. Apprenticeships transmitted knowledge and practice from one generation to the next. More recently, health work has been structured into highly organized systems led by professionals with advanced education and certification following approved standards of practice.

For many people today, the term "health worker" conjures up an image of a doctor or nurse, dressed in a white or green coat, providing advanced care in a sanitized hospital setting. Yet for the overwhelming bulk of the world's people, these professionals are inaccessible and unaffordable. Doctors and nurses overwhelmingly dominate the hierarchy of medical systems in nearly all countries, but they make up a small part of the total health workforce in both rich and poor countries. Instead, a diverse set of frontline workers provides the bulk of health services, linking people in communities to health knowledge, health technologies, and health services.

Fundamental to meeting a family's health needs is access to a motivated, skilled, and supported health worker. A frontline health worker bridges the gap between the potential for health and its realization. Breakthroughs in science and technology may be spectacular. But they sit on the shelf unless people can get to health workers who can help translate these advances into better health.

This chapter addresses the desire of every community to have access to motivated and competent health workers. This is the fundamental

❝ **The goal for every community is access to a motivated and competent health worker, backed by sustainable national health systems**

aim of all sustainable national health systems. And in hard-pressed countries experiencing health crises, the rapid mobilization of community-based workers is an immediate priority for urgent action. That is why this chapter focuses on health workers at the frontlines in communities around the world. (It does not attempt to cover all aspects of community and national health systems, which have been covered elsewhere.[1])

Workers at the frontlines

People are the primary producers of health for themselves and their families. They undertake most health-related activities—food and nutrition, hygiene and sanitation, healthy or risky behavior. Health workers link themselves and their families to wider systems of knowledge, technologies, and services. This human interaction of workers with people is the catalyst of health production.

Who is a health worker? All workers protecting and improving the health of individuals and populations, with functions ranging from clinical care to prevention and promotion and policy advocacy (figure 2.1). According to the WHO, "human resources, the different kinds of clinical and non-clinical staff who make each individual and public health intervention happen, are the most important of the health system inputs. The performance of health care systems depends ultimately on the knowledge, skills, and motivation of the people responsible for delivering services."[2] This comprehensive definition encompasses the full spectrum of health workers and their roles, function, and arrangements.

Using this definition, the health workforce varies greatly in its composition from country to country. Health workers may be formally or informally organized, paid or unpaid, practicing modern or

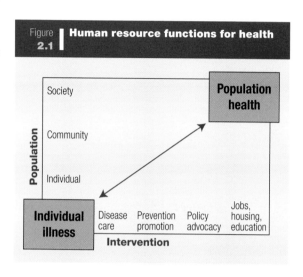

Figure 2.1 | Human resource functions for health

traditional medicine, and generalized or specialized in their scope of practice. The balance and distribution of health workers across categories and in terms of gender, skills, preventative or curative focus, private or public sector employment, and geographic location are all important workforce attributes. Ensuring the appropriate composition of worker teams is often more important than individual roles and skills.

Workers at the frontline of health care display enormous diversity worldwide. Village health clinics, intensive care units, local pharmacy shops, and hospital emergency rooms are all the frontlines of health production in diverse communities—urban and rural, rich and poor, tropical and temperate.

The frontline of health production can be depicted as a pyramid (figure 2.2). At the base is the interface of people and workers, with the family caregiver as the most important provider. One step removed are informal and traditional workers—numerous and near families. Community health workers, usually recruited and trained locally in both public and private systems, are also a strong

Figure 2.2 | **Family workers at the base of the pyramid—professionals at the top**

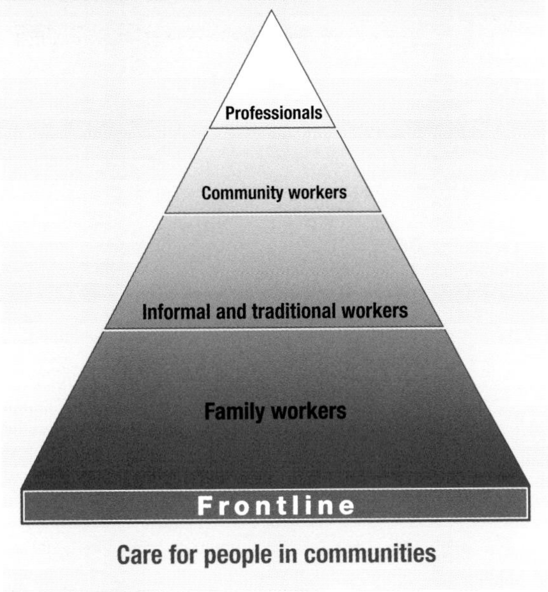

- Professionals
- Community workers
- Informal and traditional workers
- Family workers

Frontline

Care for people in communities

> **The education and power of women are among the most important determinants of health**

While the care economy is often unrecognized and undervalued, the United Nations Development Programme estimates that nonmonetized activities, if valued as market transactions, would generate another $16 trillion of global product—adding 70 percent to current estimates of world economic output.[4] Estimates suggest that two-thirds of this $16 trillion comes from the invisible contribution of women. Because women do the most important frontline work of promoting health and health care, the education and power of women are among the most important determinants of health.[5]

HIV/AIDS has compelled recognition of family caregivers in hard-hit countries. If not themselves ill, women, the elderly, and even children are absorbing the huge care burden of the epidemic (box 2.1). Women and girls are expected to assume these nurturing roles in most societies. And where adult women are absent, the elderly are assuming caregiving and family earning roles vacated by sick adults. Children—especially teenage girls—grow up assuming adult responsibilities before they become adults. Orphans are making continuing demands on family and community members.

HIV/AIDS is also exerting enormous pressures on community-based mutual care and support systems—which link invisible family workers. While different community mechanisms exist, in most societies community members provide each other with psychosocial support and have various means of sharing the burden of caring for the sick in the community. Many community-based programs of governments and nongovernmental organizations rely on these community systems to facilitate care. As long as these programs contribute financially, strengthen skill development, and do not make overwhelming

presence, linked to vocational workers and advanced professionals in district and national systems. All these workers constitute a nation's health workforce.

"Invisible" workers—in families

In a health crisis, it is most often family members—by culture or tradition, women—who ease pain and suffering, offer physical care and nurturing, and provide comfort and support. They are "invisible" because they are often taken for granted, with no formal training, and invariably unpaid.

This invisible health worker often assumes other unpaid household responsibilities—collecting water, preparing food, caring for children, and doing the cleaning. This work adds up. Of all productive activities by women, the care economy may constitute as much as 70 percent of women's unpaid economic activity.[3]

> **“** **The closest and most numerous health workers outside the household are informal and traditional**

Box 2.1 | The invisible workforce

"I thought HIV/AIDS was the concern of doctors, but later I discovered...it has become our problem and concern."
— *A community counselor, Sudan (HelpAge 2003, p.16)*

The typical caregiver of a person living with HIV or AIDS is not wearing a white coat or a stethoscope. Increasingly, she is a wife or parent forced to take on the three roles of caregiver, sole income earner, and homemaker. With the HIV/AIDS pandemic overwhelming the capacity of health systems worldwide and increasing the strain on already limited human resources for health, families are providing health care to people living with HIV/AIDS and doing what used to be the domain of formal health workers. This new generation of informal caregivers

is largely unpaid—and often invisible, especially in rural areas.

These caregivers provide vital support to their family members affected by HIV/AIDS, performing three major tasks. They assist with the needs of daily living. They help with health care. And they provide moral support. The burden of caring around the HIV/AIDS epidemic disproportionately affects women as society's traditional caregivers.

Yet HIV/AIDS prevention and care programs have not adequately acknowledged the value and needs of the invisible health workforce. In the face of death, disability, illness, and grief, the burden of caring for patients affected with HIV/AIDS causes many stresses. Providing support to care providers is thus key to preventing burnout and reducing stress and anxiety. In Vietnam the

Vietnam Women's Union has helped caregivers form clubs to discuss the impact of HIV/AIDS on their lives and seek support and advice.

As knowledge bearers, educators, and moral guides, informal caregivers make up a vast pool of human capital that can be harnessed in HIV/AIDS prevention and care. Since providing care places significant burdens on family and community members— including the removal from paid jobs because of caring duties— informal caregivers can benefit from programs that help to meet their material needs and offset the financial and time stresses they face in providing care. Such support can be provided through credit programs, basic ration provision, social security benefits, and other social protection measures.

Source: Armstrong 2000; Saengtienchai and Knodel 2001; HelpAge 2003.

---

demands on uncompensated time, they can tap the potential of community assets without further burdening a community's already stretched resources.

Informal and traditional workers

The closest and most numerous health workers outside the household are informal and traditional. Informal workers are an assortment of independent practitioners, pharmacy shop operators, birth attendants, and others. They subscribe to various therapeutic theories, often in combination with allopathic schools of treatment.

Few are professionally educated or formally employed, though many may be described as small business operators. Most receive payment for service—in kind or in fees or in reciprocal exchange. The scope of their practice may be narrow, as for traditional birth attendants, or broad, as for rural medical practitioners who assume the role of primary physicians in villages and pharmacy shop managers who sell a wide range of medicines to address client symptoms.

Traditional healers—herbalists, shamans, ayurvedics, homeopaths, bonesetters, faith healers—

❝ In many parts of the world, informal and traditional healers are the first line of care beyond the family

follow traditional theories of disease causation and therapy. Sometimes traditional theory is blended with modern medicine. Most healers are informally organized, though China and India have well-structured and well-financed systems supported by the state. They too are paid in kind, in fees, or in reciprocal exchange. The scope of their practice can also be either narrow or broad. Bone-setters are very specialized, while generalist Indian ayurvedic practitioners teach an entire way of life—including diet, exercise, lifestyle, and mental outlook.

In many parts of the world, informal and traditional healers are the first line of care beyond the family. In South Asia traditional birth attendants may be found in every village. India has more than one million rural traditional practitioners.[6] Africa also has an abundance of informal and traditional workers. A majority of people in Uganda, Tanzania, Benin, Rwanda, and Ethiopia use traditional medicine,[7] the first stop for medical advice or treatment for most Africans.[8,9] Patients with tuberculosis in Malawi were found to visit traditional healers for four weeks before seeking care in the formal medical system.[10]

The reasons for preferring and relying on these workers in poor communities are straightforward. They offer physical access to services not provided by modern systems, and they are present in communities unserved or underserved by the formal health care system. The density of informal and traditional workers in marginal regions can be many times greater than workers of the formal system.[11]

Traditional workers also offer cultural compatibility. They are generally long-standing members of the community, with a shared language and culture easing communications. There is also social responsiveness. Public services are sometimes

perceived as impersonal, unfriendly, and cumbersome because of long waiting times. But informal and traditional workers keep no formal office hours, spend more time with patients, and pay home visits. Their fees are also likely to be lower than those in the formal system, private or public. But among their numbers are charlatans and unscrupulous practitioners, often unregulated and sometimes dangerous.

The policy challenge is to build on the strengths of traditional practitioners while using education and collaboration with the formal health sector to minimize their weaknesses. Training programs for traditional practitioners and opportunities for health professionals to learn traditional practices, such as those in Kenya and Zimbabwe, are means of improving the effectiveness of traditional workers.[12]

Community health workers

Community health workers are associated with the Alma Ata primary health care movement. They provide basic health services and promote the key principles of primary health care: equity, intersectoral collaboration, community involvement, and appropriate technology.[13] The WHO underscored that community health workers should be "members of the communities where they work, should be selected by the communities, should be answerable to the communities for their activities, should be supported by the health system but not necessarily a part of its organization, and have a shorter training than professional workers."[14]

Community health workers long preceded the primary care movement and will continue far beyond it. Workers serving their communities have extended effective services throughout Asia, Africa, and Latin America. Among community health workers, there is considerable variation in

❝ In Brazil community health agents care for 93 million people across the country

work scope, training, and responsibilities (table 2.1). Often female and briefly trained, community health workers provide considerable coverage in countries with populations ranging from 100 to 1,000 people per worker. Although some workers are volunteers, most receive modest stipends. Whether voluntary or salaried, community health workers are in the public health system and in private and not-for-profit health programs.

Community workers have been deployed for general primary care as well as categorical priority programs. BRAC, a Bangladeshi nongovernmental organization, has a long-standing program of *shasta shabikas* (village workers for primary care) linked to its village-based development programs. But for a national oral rehydration therapy campaign, it recruited, trained, and salaried an additional vertically structured cadre of village workers that systematically covered the entire country. And its DOTS program against tuberculosis is a partly categorical and partly integrated program, with a special incentive scheme and dedicated laboratory services, linked to generalist *shasta shabikas* in villages. BRAC shows that community health workers can help deliver primary care, categorical programs, or a combination of the two.

In Brazil community health agents, created by the ministry of health to address the primary health care needs of marginal populations, care for 93 million people across the country.[15] Community health agents, local residents in the areas in which they work, cover 150 families in rural areas or 250 families in urban areas. Instructors or supervisors are most often nurses that reside in the local community, coach, and provide technical support. The program has shaped new referral

Table 2.1	Community health workers in Asia			
Country	**Type of worker**	**Duration of training**	**Percentage female**	**Number trained (thousands)**
India	Village health guide	3 months	25	417
Indonesia	Health cadre	3 days	100	1,800
Myanmar	Community health worker	4 weeks	5	36
	Ten-household health worker	7 days	90	42
Nepal	Female village health volunteer	12 days; 3 day yearly refresher	100	32
Sri Lanka	Volunteer health worker	6 hours	66	100

Note: Data are as of 1991 for Indonesia, 1993 for Sri Lanka, and 1994 for India, Myanmar, and Nepal.
Source: WHO Regional Office for South-East Asia 1996.

systems, enabled communities to participate in planning and performance evaluations, and fortified linkages between local communities, local health services, and state and federal actors.

Across Africa community health workers have fulfilled generalist health functions, specialist health roles in such areas as nutrition, reproductive health, and malaria control, and wider roles as community advocates and change agents. Evidence suggests that these workers have increased coverage of a range of services over the last 30 years.[16] Yet the effectiveness of community health worker programs on the continent has often been constrained by a lack of government support, the inattention to primary health care, and the reduced role of community health workers in national health care systems, particularly during political transitions.[17] A renewal of community health worker programs—better designed, managed, monitored, and evaluated, with greater support and supervision and more community

❝ Worker patterns limit—or open—possibilities for greater efficiency and effectiveness

participation and ownership—could help to meet the challenges of collapsing health systems, rising disease burdens, and departing professionals.

Professional, associate, and nonmedical workers
The most technically advanced health workers are health professionals—doctors, nurses, dentists, pharmacists, midwives, psychologists, health service managers, and others. They usually have tertiary education, and most countries have formal methods of certifying their qualifications. Technical hierarchy means that these professionals are invariably the senior-most workers in health teams and systems. When mobilized effectively, they can be outstanding leaders of health teams.

Vocational or auxiliary workers are "associate professionals" who support or substitute for university-trained professionals. They include medical, nursing and midwifery assistants, clinical officers, dental aides, physiotherapists, and laboratory technicians. In many countries, rich and poor, auxiliaries are the most numerous type of health worker. Mostly based in clinical and hospital facilities, they can also be assigned to rural health facilities in communities.

Several studies show that auxiliary workers can assume many of the functions of professionals, such as the full range of diagnostic and therapeutic services, including anaesthesia and surgery.[18] They also serve frequently as health leaders in communities, especially where doctors or nurses are hesitant to work.[19]

Nonmedical workers—accountants, drivers, and cleaners—make the health system work. Although their training and skills are not specific to health or medical care, health systems would not function without them.

Worker patterns
In addition to family caregivers are five groups of health workers: informal and traditional workers, community workers, associate professionals, professionals, and nonmedical workers. They encompass the full spectrum of health workers that can be applied across countries. While some functions can be matched to each group, there is also considerable duplication among groups, as well as possible delegation of even the most complex tasks to less formally educated workers.

National patterns vary greatly. A full census of all health workers in a single country is not readily available, but a study in Bangladesh and a recent WHO sample survey of health facilities found extraordinary diversity in national worker patterns (figure 2.3).[20] Chad illustrates the spectrum: few physicians and pharmacists in relation to much more numerous nurses and midwives. The largest groups of workers: auxiliary nurses and midwives, and others. Health workers in Chad are mostly men, in contrast to the female predominance in most other countries.

Despite limited information gathered from the sample surveys, workforce patterns in Bangladesh, Chad, Côte d'Ivoire, Mozambique, and Sri Lanka underscore the variability in national workforces. Across the five countries physicians, nurses, and midwives range from 19 percent of the workforce in Bangladesh to 73 percent in Sri Lanka. In most countries, women dominate in nursing and midwifery positions while men dominate in medicine.

Worker patterns are important because they limit—or open—possibilities for greater efficiency

Figure
2.3 | **Sample survey of national workforce patterns**

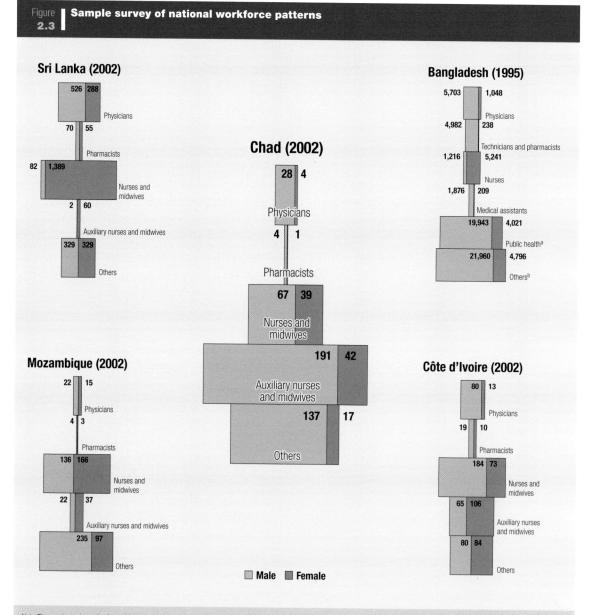

Sri Lanka (2002)

526	288
	Physicians
70	55
	Pharmacists
82	1,389
	Nurses and midwives
2	60
	Auxiliary nurses and midwives
329	329
	Others

Chad (2002)

28	4
	Physicians
4	1
	Pharmacists
67	39
	Nurses and midwives
191	42
	Auxiliary nurses and midwives
137	17
	Others

Bangladesh (1995)

5,703	1,048
	Physicians
4,982	238
	Technicians and pharmacists
1,216	5,241
	Nurses
1,876	209
	Medical assistants
19,943	4,021
	Public health[a]
21,960	4,796
	Others[b]

Mozambique (2002)

22	15
	Physicians
4	3
	Pharmacists
136	166
	Nurses and midwives
22	37
	Auxiliary nurses and midwives
235	97
	Others

Côte d'Ivoire (2002)

80	13
	Physicians
19	10
	Pharmacists
184	73
	Nurses and midwives
65	106
	Auxiliary nurses and midwives
80	84
	Others

■ **Male** ■ **Female**

Note: The numbers shown for Chad, Côte d'Ivoire, Mozambique, and Sri Lanka indicate the total number of health workers interviewed from the health facilities selected for the survey. The numbers shown for Bangladesh indicate the results of personnel data collected from all health establishments under the Ministry of Health.

a. Sanitary inspector, health inspector, assistant health inspector, health assistant.

b. Primarily cleaning, sweeping, and clerical jobs.

Source: WHO 2004, except for Bangladesh, from Hossain and Begum 1998.

and effectiveness. Investments in worker training may be concentrated on fewer professionals or on briefly trained community health workers. Some worker functions can be either substituted or delegated. Some are better performed by teams rather than individuals.

Although there is no one optimal national pattern, most configurations show room for improvement. For example, the ratio of only one nurse for every three doctors in Latin America severely constrains efficiency improvements by making it difficult to delegate from more to less expensive personnel. The male bias in the formal health sector in Bangladesh and Chad compromises women's access to culturally appropriate health services.

Workers in community systems

All workers want to serve their communities. But many are not properly assigned. Others receive training inappropriate to the tasks before them. Many may also suffer from weak support from district or national systems for legal/regulatory frameworks, information, supervision, or the availability of drugs and supplies. Not infrequently, the reporting line of workers is to distant headquarters rather than to the communities they serve. The misfit between servicing community clients and being accountable to headquarters can result in poor worker performance—and lead to irregular worker hours, absenteeism, and a lack of courtesy and responsiveness to clients.

Core strategies for workers at the frontline should thus seek to strengthen the dedication, service, and effectiveness of workers by increasing community participation and control—reinforced by national and district level legal/regulatory frameworks,

supervision, technical support, and financing. Workforce strategies for sustainable community systems should aim for aligning services and accountability, channeling appropriate support to communities, and expanding community financing.

Aligning service with accountability

A key strategy for strengthening community workers is to increase their accountability to local clients and authorities. Stronger accountability to the community would compel them to engage with community leaders and organizations, such as traditional chiefs, religious leaders, elected officials, community-based organizations, women's associations, youth and citizen groups, and NGOs. Those leaders and organizations should participate in the design, implementation, and evaluation of health programs. In some communities, village or neighborhood health committees provide such input. The World Bank, in its *2004 World Development Report: Making Services Work for Poor People*, argues for better balancing central and community accountability to improve the responsiveness of public services to the needs of the poor (figure 2.4).

Worker satisfaction and performance also are enhanced when workers are recruited from and trained to perform functions most appropriate to the community—and when they join locally-based teams that work together to serve the community. Local recruitment and assignment increase social and cultural compatibility and worker efficiency (box 2.2). Absenteeism, for example, is greatly reduced by having workers recruited and assigned locally.[21] Local recruitment and assignment also enhance the sustainability of community work: rural retention can be career-long. The key to retaining workers in rural

❝❝ **Worker satisfaction and performance are enhanced when workers are recruited from the community**

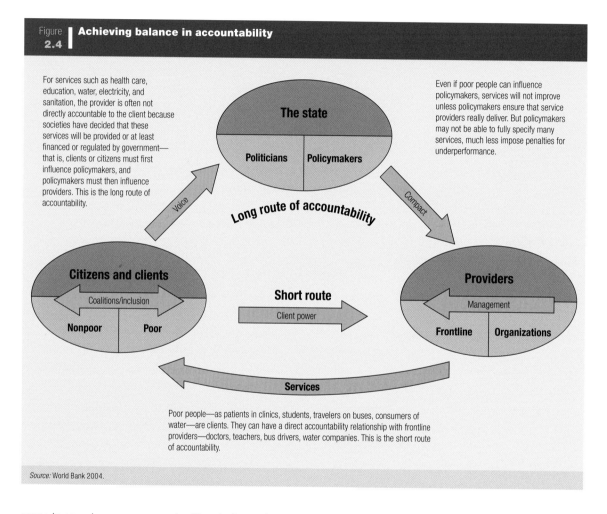

Figure 2.4 | **Achieving balance in accountability**

For services such as health care, education, water, electricity, and sanitation, the provider is often not directly accountable to the client because societies have decided that these services will be provided or at least financed or regulated by government—that is, clients or citizens must first influence policymakers, and policymakers must then influence providers. This is the long route of accountability.

Even if poor people can influence policymakers, services will not improve unless policymakers ensure that service providers really deliver. But policymakers may not be able to fully specify many services, much less impose penalties for underperformance.

The state

Politicians | Policymakers

Voice

Compact

Long route of accountability

Citizens and clients

Coalitions/inclusion

Nonpoor | Poor

Short route

Client power

Providers

Management

Frontline | Organizations

Services

Poor people—as patients in clinics, students, travelers on buses, consumers of water—are clients. They can have a direct accountability relationship with frontline providers—doctors, teachers, bus drivers, water companies. This is the short route of accountability.

Source: World Bank 2004.

areas is ensuring career opportunities similar to those available to workers in more privileged locations.

Training should also orient workers to local communities. Knowledge and experience of community health concerns and local realities are crucial. Community-oriented curricula ensure that trainees acquire the skills most needed. These include nonmedical technical skills—such as communication, relationship building, and participatory work approaches. Basing medical and nursing education and short-term training programs in communities—and including community rotations in training placements—enhance the relevance of training and improve worker retention. Innovative training programs, like the University of Transkei's in South Africa, have incorporated community representatives in exercises. Others have fostered partnerships among educational institutions, national health programs, and local communities.[22]

Community accountability must be balanced by support and reinforcement from the district and national levels

---

Box 2.2 | Recruiting locally is the most important first step

The government of Thailand has had great success in improving equitable access to health care throughout the country over the last four decades. In 1977, 46 percent of outpatient visits were to urban provincial hospitals, only 29 percent to rural health centers. Over the next 30 years, a concerted program of rural health development reversed that trend. By 2000 only 18 percent of outpatient visits were to urban provincial hospitals, and visits to rural health centers had almost doubled—to 46 percent.

Attracting and training health professionals from rural populations has been an important part of Thailand's success. The ministry of public health recruits nurses, midwives, junior sanitarians, and other paramedics and trains them locally in nursing and public health colleges around the country. It then assigns them placements in their hometowns on graduation, and licenses them for service in the public sector alone. All this has helped to create a strong core of local health workers in Thailand.

Thailand's local recruiting efforts have been mostly positive, showing how countries can address the inequitable distribution of health workers. But to have the greatest impact, rural recruitment programs must be in a wider context of support for rural health personnel. That means improving rural health infrastructure. Offering access to training and career advancement opportunities to rural workers. Providing attractive financial incentives, including hardship allowances for rural service. And perhaps most important, making a long-term political commitment to supporting health workers and investing in the national public health care system.

Source: Wibulpolprasert and Pengpaibon 2003.

Worker teams should be built to match community needs. Costa Rica's Basic Health Attention Teams have revitalized the country's primary health care system and reduced disparities in coverage between urban and rural populations. Located in small clinics or peripheral facilities in the country's 90 health areas, teams are responsible for a community's physical and social needs. Each team, with a doctor, nurse, and technician, is responsible for around 4,000 people.[23] Never alone, the workers are always backed by the supervision, technical support, and drugs and supplies of team systems. The community workers identify individuals and families at risk, provide home care for certain illnesses, and provide referrals to second- and third-level facilities.

Special outreach to marginal communities is also needed. These include slum dwellers, immigrants, refugees, commercial sex workers, and drug addicts. Effective strategies to reach these populations depend on their peers, the only ones to have access and credibility to reach out to stigmatized and ostracized communities. Look at the way HIV-positive people have organized themselves and moved the policy and action agenda. And peer workers among them have increased access, impact, and accountability.

Channeling appropriate support

Community accountability must be balanced by support and reinforcement from the district and national levels in leadership, coordination, and the replenishment of essential drugs

❝ Community financing can improve access to care and provide financial protection against catastrophic health care costs

and supplies. Unsupported by higher levels, community programs are difficult to sustain.

Particularly important is the sensitivity of management to class and gender dimensions. Improving the social standing and professional esteem of frontline workers can improve recruitment and motivation. Addressing the special challenges that female workers face can also improve performance. They consistently report competing demands of work with domestic responsibilities, cultural taboos and constraints, discrimination, physical threats, sexual harassment, and separation from families in remote locations.

Success stories in countries as diverse as Iran, Brazil, and Costa Rica all suggest that it is possible to adopt integrated management systems involving community organizations, local administrative structures, and national systems. Such systems balance community participation and control with central leadership and operational structures to support frontline health workers. Yet many countries undergoing health sector reform are currently struggling with this balance between community action and national systems.

Decentralizing responsibility for worker hiring, placement, and management from national to district and community levels profoundly affects workers who require support to serve their communities. In theory at least, local recruitment, training, and accountability have many positive aspects. But decentralization also raises worker concerns over job insecurity, inequities in salaries among different workers for the same work, and insufficient continuing education and career development opportunities. Some of these unsettling developments have escalated to union protests and worker strikes.

Of course, decentralizing worker management must be preceded or accompanied by decentralizing financial and management capacity to communities and local government, including the administration of public expenditures. There are many cases where budgetary ceilings, financial regulations, or legislative controls put in place before decentralization have not been updated. In Kenya, for example, donor funds are paralyzed because administrative procedures for decentralized fiscal management have not been finalized. Sequencing and coordinating decentralization is thus essential.

Expanding community financing

It is hard to sustain health systems based on volunteerism and donations. Community health financing has been advanced to counter the limitations. Examples include the Bamako Initiative for revolving drug funds and Vimo SEWA's affordable health insurance for the poor (box 2.3).

Evidence shows that community financing can improve access to care and provide financial protection against catastrophic health care costs.[24] It can also increase the sense of accountability of health workers and health services to the community. But not all community financing programs have been successful in their functions and sustainability, particularly in very poor communities. The poverty of many communities, the small risk pool of insurance, and the fluctuations and volatility in costs are among the reasons for failure.

Community systems invariably require cofinancing from district or national level insurance systems. Cofinancing is necessary to expand the risk pool and to protect for fiscal fluctuations. Technical, administrative, and financial support are also essential for the survival of community health insurance.

❝❝ Community systems invariably require cofinancing from district or national level insurance systems

---

Box 2.3 | SEWA's community financing

Vimo SEWA, established by the Self-Employed Women's Association (SEWA) in Gujarat, India, has been proving health insurance to members and their families since 1992. It is run by local women with the support of a full-time staff and a team of experienced medical, public health, and insurance experts. Under the most popular policy, an annual premium of 85 rupees—22.5 rupees for health insurance, with the remainder for life and asset insurance—provides coverage for a maximum of 2,000 rupees a year in case of hospitalization. Members are eligible for reimbursement whether they choose private for-profit, private nonprofit, or public health services.

Claims are verified by a SEWA employee, a consultant physician, and an insurance committee. Vimo SEWA has nearly 103,000 members from both urban and rural Gujarat.

Four key factors facilitated Vimo SEWA's growth and success.

- Nesting Vimo SEWA in a larger membership-based organization encouraged collaboration and participation among members— and provided infrastructure and human resource support.
- Premiums and benefits were based on data determined in collaboration with the Government Insurance Company, and any increase in premiums was gradual.

- Technical and (small but reliable) financial support from development partners enabled Vimo SEWA to market its insurance plan among a largely rural and illiterate population.
- A flexible and dynamic management plan allowed Vimo SEWA to adapt in response to member needs and external evaluations.

The challenge to SEWA's sustainability is to expand the insurance pool by linking such microsystems into larger national systems that spreads risks, provides fiscal stability, and systematically expands coverage linked to affordability and health safety.

Source: Chatterjee and Ranson 2003.

Management capacity will need to be strengthened and effective linkages between local schemes and formal health financing systems enacted. When insurance-based or tax-financed universal health insurance is not affordable, the combination of community and national financing is appropriate.

Mobilizing health workers

Many countries today, unfortunately, do not have the option to build sustainable health systems over years. Contemporary health crises are so severe that unless the tide is turned there can be no prospect of idealized health systems. Rapid, urgent, dramatic actions are imperative for many countries in crisis.

Organizing emergency responses requires the urgent mobilization, training, and deployment of workers. Yet the societies requiring an urgent response are the same ones already suffering from eroding health systems and severe worker shortages. To mobilize workers in these settings, the mass of invisible workers, informal and traditional workers, community health workers, and associate professionals must be harnessed. Relying on professionals is simply ineffective and unrealistic for these countries.

Worker mobilizations should focus on specific targets or goals. China's massive mobilization of more than a million barefoot doctors and three million rural health aides from the 1950s to 1970s

" **Choosing between a general and selective mobilization approach will depend on the context, needs, and political priorities**

Box 2.4 | Smallpox eradication in India: Tensions and harmony with the health system

Perhaps one of the grandest health efforts in the 20th century was the eradication of smallpox. How does mobilizing vast cadres of workers for such campaigns strengthen or weaken health systems? Here is one historian's perspective that focuses on the tensions and harmony of smallpox workers in India.

In 1968 the government of India agreed to join the global eradication effort by making smallpox vaccination a priority, deploying workers, and collaborating with the WHO in Geneva and in its South-East Asia Regional Office. A special smallpox eradication unit was set up in New Delhi to liaise with the WHO and state officials for vaccination, registration, and disease surveillance. But the commitment of personnel was variable, and many workers did not subscribe

to the view that smallpox would be eradicated through a concerted nationwide campaign of surveillance, containment, and ring vaccination.

So, a special workforce was developed, involving a core of epidemiologists hired by the WHO deputed to the Indian government. The vertically structured program trained new vaccinators, supervisors, paramedical workers, local bureaucrats, medical students, and, most strikingly, influential local leaders. This multifaceted workforce allowed the federal and state governments, backed by the WHO, to carry out intensive searches for smallpox, isolating cases and systematically breaking chains of variola transmission.

The special program eradicated smallpox, but it also generated many tensions. The exceptional

attention—higher work and travel allowances and privileged access to fellowships and training opportunities for smallpox workers—caused resentment among regular health staff. More complicated were positive legacies of target-driven working habits versus the costly consequence of having to continue to pay and absorb workers recruited after smallpox was eradicated.

A major lesson is the critical importance of workers drawn from localities, workers able to provide invaluable information on their communities. Another lesson is not to oversimplify the interaction of vertical programs and horizontal health systems—but to recognize and cope with tensions and to search for synergies that can achieve and sustain program targets and system goals.

Source: Bhattacharya 2004.

allowed for primary health coverage of previously underserved rural communities. Raising life expectancy and reducing infant mortality and crude death rates improved the health of more than 500 million people in communities across China.[25]

Beyond expanding primary services, mobilizations can also concentrate on disease control, as demonstrated by immunization campaigns and smallpox eradication (box 2.4). Choosing between a general and selective mobilization approach will depend on the local context, needs, and political priorities, often

involving domestic and foreign actors. Both options have yielded important successes and neither is automatically better or worse.[26]

The key to successful mobilization? When health workers are organized, supported, and energized, the accomplishments can be great. When they are fragmented, torn apart by multiple tasks, or demotivated, mobilization efforts will fail. The fragmentation of worker efforts can be worsened when separate mobilizations have disconnected training programs or competing incentive payments. The goals, tasks, and incentives for general and

> **The challenge is to strengthen worker systems, rather than fragment or vitiate the workforce**

priority programs should be harmonized—both for similar workers and for separate cadres of workers.

Three strategies for mobilizing health workers for urgent action: targeting all workers, aligning worker incentives, and gaining political commitment.

Targeting all workers

Experience repeatedly confirms that confining urgent health action to the health system is insufficient. All domestic actors should be mobilized, greatly expanding beyond the traditional boundaries of the health sector. The actors extend beyond government to include business and civil society. Imaginative engagement has included the entertainment industry, local and street theatre, the military, women's associations, sporting groups, religious organizations, and traditional healers (box 2.5). Wholesale imports of foreign workers can be both ineffective and expensive.

The child survival revolution spearheaded by UNICEF in the 1980s employed "social mobilization" to engage diverse actors for growth monitoring, oral rehydration therapy, breastfeeding, and immunizations. Depending heavily on informal and traditional community workers, the polio eradication campaign mobilized 10 million workers over 36 months to immunize 600 million children in 100 countries (box 2.6). The effort had five key elements—identifying available human resources, adapting tasks to match the available skills, ensuring political advocacy for social mobilization, improving management, and providing effective technical assistance.

Effective mobilizations must ensure that career prospects are available to workers once the program has ended. With the training and experience they gain, these workers are a resource to further other health goals beyond the immediate ones for which

| Box 2.5 | **Ethiopia's military—mobilizing against HIV/AIDS** |

After a 1996 survey among army blood donors revealed an HIV/AIDS prevalence rate of 6 percent, the Ethiopian Defense Force command gave HIV/AIDS control a high priority.

To spearhead the response, HIV/AIDS committees were established at all levels of the military (from the ministry to battalion command level), including ground and air forces. Measures to curb HIV/AIDS integrated AIDS programming into all army activities.

What distinguished this approach from most other military AIDS programs is having responsibility for controlling HIV a part of the core activities of the command at every level, not delegating it to the health corps alone.

Seroprevalence surveys in 2001 showed that the prevalence of HIV infections had not increased, even with a fivefold increase in the size of the armed forces.

Source: Lieutenant General (Retired) Gebre Tsadkan Gebretensae.

they were trained. Too often however, the records of these workers are not kept after the program is over and their skills and training are lost to future efforts. Resources are required to support worker transitions into their next jobs—creating permanent positions with definitive career paths for emergency workers.

Aligning worker incentives

Mobilizations often have the dual goal of achieving specific targets while building coherent and effective health systems. The challenge is to strengthen the workforce, rather than fragment or weaken it. Ambitious targets may overwhelm worker capacity and force tradeoffs with other priority tasks. Under these circumstances, workers can be torn apart by competing priorities. Strategies for alignment of incentives and synergy should thus be central

" Popular mobilization of workers can be harnessed to strengthen, not weaken, health systems

---

Box 2.6 | Mobilizing workers to eradicate polio

By 2000 the Global Polio Eradication Partnership was mobilizing more than 10 million volunteers and health workers each year to immunize 600 million children with 2 billion doses of vaccine in nearly 100 countries. As a result, by 2003 polio had been eliminated from all but 6 countries, and the incidence of the disease came down from an estimated 350,000 cases a year to 700.

The initiative used a five-part strategy to mobilize and train 10 million workers over 36 months to deliver polio vaccines to every child in the world.

1. **Identify the available human resources and skills.** The broad range of human resources that could be mobilized was identified, including skilled health workers, literate volunteers, and illiterate volunteers, from the public sector, private companies, individuals, and nongovernmental agencies, both national and international.

2. **Adapt strategies and tasks to skill levels.** Having identified the minimum skill level available, the strategy or intervention was modified accordingly. In southern Sudan, for example, all training materials were adapted to a largely illiterate population, and local wisdom was incorporated into the service delivery strategy. In the absence of electricity and refrigerators, local approaches to preserving meat were used to keep vaccines cold.

3. **Ensure political advocacy for social mobilization.** A tremendous investment in political advocacy made it possible to access the human resources in other government sectors and leverage the public communications capacity to ensure massive volunteer participation. In all countries, the tasks were designed to minimize the time demand on volunteers.

4. **Improve management.** As workers were mobilized

to deliver vaccines on a massive scale globally, simple management tools and strategies ensured optimum efficiency in the use of resources. Particular attention went to cascading training, local microplanning, and tracking the impact and quality of service delivery.

5. **Provide technical assistance.** With more countries planning for polio immunization days, demand surged for WHO's technical assistance, especially for project planning. At the peak of the initiative, WHO deployed 1,500 technical staff globally, the vast majority of them nationals, many expected to return to national service. Efforts were made to ensure that the recruitment and remuneration of these staff were negotiated with country governments in accord with their broader staffing policies and goals.

Source: Bruce Aylward, coordinator of the WHO's Global Polio Eradication Initiative.

---

to the planning and implementation of high priority mobilization efforts. This is a major challenge for such efforts as WHO's 3 by 5 Initiative.[27]

Emerging priority programs must pursue every opportunity to strengthen existing programs.[28] Shorter term mobilization and ongoing health system development can be coordinated by

sharing information and schedules, closely managing domestic and international actors, and matching short-term training to the career development of workers. Synergies can also be captured by increasing the overall pool of workers through training, skill development, and field experience, enhancing public trust and

> ❝ **National mobilizations should build up from the community, but they should also reach downwards to communities**

public demand for all services, and improving the training and management of all workers.[29]

Workers should be seen as an investment for a shared human infrastructure. Resource competition between priority programs and health system development can cause friction.[30] Diverting resources to high priority programs can weaken systems development, but high priority programs can also mobilize or even enhance incremental funding. Finances for priority programs and general system budgets should be transparent, with the population's health as the deciding factor in allocations. People benefit little if controlling one disease leads to the neglect of other equally lethal diseases, yielding no net health gain or even health reversal.

Conducting health system impact assessments before mobilizing workers, along with ongoing monitoring and evaluation, can improve the coherence of different health programs. Tuberculosis and leprosy control programs have produced useful frameworks and planning tools for assessing program impact and strengthening other systems.[31] Specific to local situations, the assessments should include program timetables, geographic coverage of remote communities, special training of multifunctional workers, and employing workers beyond the end of the priority program. With constant monitoring and adaptation, early difficulties can trigger responsive measures to reduce worker tension, program conflict, and duplications and gaps in services.

Gaining political commitment

Experience demonstrates that worker mobilization is not an isolated technical action. Indeed, terms such as social mobilization or popular mobilization have been employed to capture the breadth of

societal engagement that must be energized to create the impetus for worker mobilization. A broader political, social, and popular base for mobilization gives workers a strong sense of mission that can be motivating, exhilarating, and deeply satisfying.

Popular mobilization of workers can also be harnessed to strengthen, not weaken, health systems. By creating additional workers, improving training for existing workers, and increasing the knowledge of the general population, health mobilizations can strengthen the overall health system. And introducing new services can build the trust of consumers in the health system and in health workers, inducing demand for other services.[32] The polio eradication initiative, for example, has been associated with higher demand for other immunization services, improving the health services infrastructure.[33]

Worker mobilizations thus merit a political commitment from the highest levels of government. Innovations by individual communities are crucial, but scattered efforts are insufficient without national leadership and commitment (box 2.7). Yes, national mobilizations should build up from the community, but they should also reach downwards to communities. Political support for workers should be translated into meeting worker priorities, thus engendering stronger motivation, dedication, skills, and supportive systems. Additional financing, coupled with political support, can ensure that resources are available for urgent mobilizations without being diverted from other workers and health promotion activities.

Conclusion

Frontline health workers are indispensable to promoting sustainable community health systems and mobilizing for medical emergencies. Although

❝ In low-income communities, informal, traditional, and community health workers are essential

Costa Rica abolished its army in 1947 so that it could—at least in theory—spend on its social and health services what other countries spend on arms and the military. Its energetic political and financial commitment to health and the health workforce have raised health indicators, improved equity, and reduced the gap in the quality of care for urban and rural dwellers. It is a model for effective and equitable health and development.

In the 1970s the Costa Rican Social Security Institute was put in charge of extending universal social security legislation and universal health care coverage. It extended health services into underserved rural and marginal urban areas, launched immunization programs, and engaged local community health providers at the front lines of the health workforce. The infectious diseases and infant diarrheas once responsible for high infant mortality rates were drastically reduced, and maternal mortality also came down. Since the early 1980s Costa Rica's national health statistics rival those of much richer industrialized countries.

In the 1990s the primary health care system was strengthened by bringing essential health services closer to the people and increasing the capacity of district-level clinics. The reforms reduced expenditures while increasing productivity. They also increased the coverage of services readily available—and patient satisfaction. Health workers around the country are mobilized in Basic Health Attention Teams (EBAIS). Delivery and access to services were also expanded through complementary mechanisms such as health worker incentives for good performance and achieving goals.

The lesson from Costa Rica's experience is clear: fostering political commitment and a national consensus on the priorities of health and social development can invigorate the health workforce and greatly improve equitable access to essential health services.

Source: Clark 2002; PAHO 2002; WHO 2003.

neither paid nor specialized, many individuals, families and communities are central in promoting health. In low-income communities, informal, traditional, and community health workers are essential, supplemented by associate professionals. Highly skilled professionals like doctors, nurses, dentists, and pharmacists are rarely the foot soldiers of community health action. But they provide links to other cadres through referral systems, and they take the lead in health system innovation. Without their leadership, it is difficult to mount major urgent programs.

Strategies for workers should steer a course between two extremes. The first extreme is a top-down elitism preoccupied with doctors and nurses in advanced tertiary care facilities. This neglects the frontline for most health production in the world's communities. The other extreme is a bottom-up romanticism of ideal villages solving any problem if only they were delegated the power to do so. But communities are neither homogeneous nor isolated. Extraordinarily diverse, they are deeply imbedded in district, national, regional, and global forces that can strengthen or weaken their efforts. Community approaches must navigate through ordinary people living in diverse communities and national authorities responsible for advancing the health of all citizens.

Notes

1. Roemer 1991; Roemer 1993; WHO 2000; World Bank 2004.
2. WHO 2000.

3. ILO 2004.
4. UNDP 1995.
5. Caldwell 1986.
6. Rohde and Viswanathan 1995.
7. Chatora 2003.
8. Fournier and Haddad 1995.
9. Pretorius 1999.
10. Brouwer and others 1998.
11. Chatora 2003.
12. JLI Africa Working Group 2004.
13. Walt 1990.
14. WHO 1987, cited in WHO 1989, p. 6.
15. Campos and others 2004.
16. Lehmann and others 2004.
17. Sanders 1992; Lehmann and others 2004.
18. Dovlo 2004.
19. Couper and others 2004.
20. Hossain and Begum 1998; WHO 2004.
21. Chaudhury and Hammer 2003.
22. Lehmann and others 2000.
23. WHO 2003.
24. Preker and others 2002; Ekman 2004.
25. Campos and others 2004.
26. Cueto 2004.
27. To get antiretroviral drugs to 3 million people living with AIDS in developing countries by 2005.
28. JLI Priority Diseases Working Group 2004.
29. Melgaard and others 1998.
30. Bhattacharya 2004.
31. Atun and others 2004; Visschedijk and Feenstra 2003; Visschedijk and others 2003.
32. JLI Priority Diseases Working Group 2004.
33. Gounder 1998.

References

Armstrong, Sue. 2000. *Caring for Carers: Managing Stress in Those Who Care for People with HIV and AIDS*. Geneva: Joint United Nations Programme on HIV/AIDS.

Atun, R. A., N. Lennox-Chhugani, F. Drobniewski, Y. A. Samyshkin, and R. J. Coker. 2004. "A Framework and Toolkit for Capturing the Communicable Disease Programmes within the Health System: Tuberculosis Control as an Illustrative Example." *European Journal of Public Health* 14 (3): 267–73.

Barrett, S. 1996. "Zimbabwe Uses All Medical Resources to Find Solutions." *AIDS Analysis Africa* 6 (1): 13.

Bhat, R. 1999. "Characteristics of Private Medical Practice in India: A Provider Perspective." *Health Policy and Planning* 14 (1): 26–37.

Bhattacharya, Sanjoy. 2004. "Uncertain Advances: A Review of the Final Phases of the Smallpox Eradication Programme in India, 1960–1980." The Wellcome Trust Centre for the History of Medicine, London.

Bossert, Thomas, Joel Beauvais, and Diana Bowser. 2000. "Decentralization of Health Systems: Preliminary Review of Four Country Case Studies." Major Applied Research 6, Technical Report 1. Partnerships for Health Reform, Bethesda, Md.

Bossert, Thomas, Mukosha Bona Chitah, Maryse Simonet, Ladslous Mwansa, Maureen Daura, Musa Mabandhala, Diana Bowser, Joseph Sevilla, Joel Beauvais, Gloria Silondwa, and Munalinga Simatele. 2000. "Decentralization of the Health System in Zambia." Major Applied Research 6, Technical Report 2. Partnerships for Health Reform, Bethesda, Md.

Brouwer, J. A., M. J. Boeree, P. Kager, C. M. Varkevisser, and A. D. Harries. 1998. "Traditional Healers and Pulmonary Tuberculosis in Malawi." *International Journal of Tuberculosis and Lung Disease* 2 (3): 231–34.

Burnett A., R. Baggaley, M. Ndovi-MacMillan, J. Sulwe, B. Hang'omba, and J. Bennett. 1999. "Caring for People with HIV in Zambia: Are Traditional Healers and Formal Health Workers Willing to Work Together?" *AIDS Care* 11 (4): 481–91.

Caldwell, James C. 1986. "Routes to Low Mortality in Poor Countries." *Population and Development Review* 12 (2): 171–220.

Campos, Francisco, José Roberto Ferreira, Maria Fátima de Souza, and Raphael Augusto Teixeira de Aguiar. 2004. "The Innovations on Human Resources Development and the Role of Community Health Workers." Joint Learning Initiative Working Paper. Universidade Federal de Minas Gerais Núcleo de Pesquisa em Saúde Coletiva, Brazil. [www.globalhealthtrust.org/].

Chatora, Rufaro. 2003. "An Overview of the Traditional Medicine Situation in the African Region." *African Health Monitor* 4 (1): 4–7.

Chatterjee, Mirai and M. Kent Ranson. 2003. "Livelihood Security through Community-Based Health Insurance in India." In Lincoln Chen, Jennifer Leaning, and Vasant Narasimhan, eds., *Global Health Challenges for Human Security*. Cambridge, Mass.: Harvard University Press.

Chaudhury, Nzamul, and Jeffrey S. Hammer. 2003. "Ghost Doctors: Absenteeism in Bangladeshi Health Facilities," Policy Research Working Paper 3065. World Bank, Washington, D.C. [Retrieved October 4, 2004, from http://econ.worldbank.org/files/27031_wps3065.pdf].

Chomitz, Kenneth M., Gunawan Setiadi, Azrul Azwar, Nusye Ismail, and Widiyarti. 1998. "What Do Doctors Want? Developing Incentives for Doctors to Serve in Indonesia's Rural and Remote Areas." Policy Research Working Paper 1888. World Bank, Washington, D.C. [www.econ.worldbank.org].

Chowdhury, A. M. R., Sadia Chowdhury, Md. Nazrul Islam, Akramul Islam, and J. Patrick Vaughan. 1997. "Control of Tuberculosis by Community Health Workers in Bangladesh." *The Lancet* 350 (9072): 169–72.

Chowdhury, Mushtaque. 2003. "Health Workforce for TB Control by DOTS: The BRAC Case." Joint Learning Initiative Working Paper. BRAC, Bangladesh. [www.globalhealthtrust.org/].

Clark, Mary. 2002. *Health Sector Reform in Costa Rica: Reinforcing a Public System*. Paper prepared for the Woodrow Wilson Center Workshops on the Politics of Education and Health Reforms, April 18–19, Washington, D.C.

Colvin M., L. Gumede, K. Grimwade, D. Maher, and D. Wilkinson. 2003. "Contribution of Traditional Healers to a Rural Tuberculosis Control Programme in Hlabisa, South Africa." *International Journal of Tuberculosis and Lung Disease* 7 (9 Suppl. 1): S86–91.

Couper, Ian, Rudi Thetard, and Colin Pfaff. 2004. "Midlevel Workers in Other Countries." Electronic Doctor Interactive. The South African Academy of Family Practice, Rural Health Initiative. Rivonia, South Africa. [Retrieved August 8, 2004, from www.edoc.co.za/modules.php?name=News&file=article&sid=512].

Cueto, Marcos. 2004. "The Origins of Primary Health Care and Selective Primary Health Care." Joint Learning Initiative Working Paper. Universidad Peruana Cayetano Heredia, Peru. [www.globalhealthtrust.org/].

de Leonardis, Ota. "Social Capital, Sociability and Health." Joint Learning Initiative Working Paper. University of Sociology and Social Research, Italy. [www.globalhealthtrust.org/].

de Waal, Alex, and Alan Whiteside. 2003. "'New Variant Famine': AIDS and Food Crisis in Southern Africa." *The Lancet* 362 (9391): 1234–37.

Diallo D., M. Koumare, A. K. Traore, R. Sanogo, and D. Coulibaly. 2003. "Collaboration between Traditional Health Practitioners and Conventional Health Practitioners: The Malian Experience." *African Health Monitor* 4 (1): 31–32.

Dieleman, Marjolein, Pham Viet Cuong, Le Vu Anh, and Tim Martineau. 2003. "Identifying Factors for Job Motivation of Rural Health Workers in North Viet Nam." *Human Resources for Health* 1 (10).

Dovlo D. 2004. "Using Mid-Level Cadres as Substitutes for Internationally Mobile Health Professionals in Africa. A desk review." *Human Resources for Health* 2 (1): 7.

Dugger, Celia W. 2004. "Deserted by Doctors, India's Poor Turn to Quacks." *New York Times*, March 25.

Egger, Dominique, Debra Lipson, and Orvill Adams. 2000. "Achieving the Right Balance: The Role of Policy-Making Processes in Managing Human Resources for Health Problems." Issues in Health Services Delivery Discussion Paper 2. World Health Organization. [www.who.int/health-services-delivery/disc_papers/Right_balance.pdf].

Ekman, Bjorn. 2004. "Community-Based Health Insurance in Low-Income Countries: A Systematic Review of the Evidence." *Health Policy and Planning* 19 (5): 249–70.

Fournier, P., and S. Haddad. 1995 "Les facteurs associés à l'utilisation des services de santé dans les pays en développement." In H. Gérard and V. Piché, eds., *Sociologie des populations*. AUPELF–UREF. Montréal: Presses de l'Université de Montréal.

Gounder, C. 1998. "The Progress of the Polio Eradication Initiative: What Prospects for Eradicating Measles." *Health Policy and Planning* 13 (3): 212–33.

Guldan, Georgia S. 1996. "Obstacles to Community Health Promotion." *Social Science and Medicine* 43 (5): 689–95.

Hadi, A. 2001. "Diagnosis of Pneumonia by Community Health Volunteers: Experience of BRAC, Bangladesh." *Tropical Doctor* 31 (2): 75–77.

———. 2003. "Management of Acute Respiratory Infections by Community Health Volunteers: Experience of Bangladesh Rural Advancement Committee (BRAC)." *Bulletin of the World Health Organization* 81 (3): 183–89.

HelpAge International and International HIV/AIDS Alliance. 2003. *Forgotten Families: Older People as Carers of Orphans and Vulnerable Children*. [www.helpage.org/].

Hossain, Belayet, and Khaleda Begum. 1998. "Survey of the Existing Health Workforce of Ministry of Health, Bangladesh." *Human Resources Development Journal* 2 (2): 109–116.

ILO (International Labour Organization). 2004. "Impact of HIV/AIDS Epidemic on Women." [Retrieved October 4, 2004, from www.ilo.org/public/english/region/eurpro/london/news/hivwom.htm].

ILO (International Labour Organization) and UNIFEM (United Nations Development Fund for Women). 2001. "Brainstorm Workshop on ILO/UNIFEM Programme: The Care Economy, HIV/AIDS and the World of Work." November 22–23, Turin, Italy.

Im-em, W., and G. Suwannarat. 2002. "Response to AIDS at Individual, Household and Community

Levels in Thailand." Draft. United Nations Research Institute for Social Development, Geneva.

Islam, Md. Akramul, Susumu Wakai, Nobukatsu Ishikawa, A. M. R. Chowdhury, and J. Patrick Vaughan. 2002. "Cost-Effectiveness of Community Health Workers in Tuberculosis Control in Bangladesh." *Bulletin of the World Health Organization* 80 (6): 445–50.

Joint Learning Initiative, Africa Working Group. 2004. "Draft Report: The Health Workforce in Africa: Challenges and Prospects." [www.globalhealthtrust.org/].

Joint Learning Initiative, Demand Working Group. 2004. "Draft Report: Health Human Resources Demand and Management: Strategies to Confront Crisis." [www.globalhealthtrust.org/].

Joint Learning Initiative, Priority Diseases Working Group. 2004. "Draft Report: Workers for Priorities in Health." [www.globalhealthtrust.org/].

Kahssay, Haile Mariam, Mary E. Taylor, and Peter A. Berman. 1998. *Community Health Workers: The Way Forward*. Geneva: World Health Organization.

Kaseje, Dan. 2003. "Promoting Community Empowerment for Effective Health and Development Action in the 21st Century." Report presented to the Rockefeller Foundation. The Tropical Institute of Community Health and Development in Africa, Nairobi.

King, R., and J. Homsy. 1997. "Involving Traditional Healers in AIDS Education and Counseling in Sub-Saharan Africa: A Review." *AIDS* 11 (Suppl. A): S217–25.

Kolehmainen-Aitken, Riita-Liisa. 2004. "Decentralization's Impact on the Health Workforce: Perspectives of Managers, Workers, and National Leaders." *Human Resources for Health* 2 (5).

Kyeyune, Primrose, Dorothy Balaba, and Jaco Homsy. 2003. "The Role of Traditional Health Practitioners in Increasing Access to HIV/AIDS Prevention and Care: The Ugandan Experience." *African Health Monitor* 4 (1): 31–32.

Lehmann, U., G. Andrews, and D. Sanders. 2000. "Change and Innovation at South African Medical Schools—An Investigation of Student Demographics, Student Support and Curriculum Innovation." Health Systems Trust Research Program. [http://new.hst.org.za/index.php].

Lehmann, Uta, Irwin Friedman, and David Sanders. 2004. "Review of the Utilization and Effectiveness of Community-Based Health Workers in Africa." Joint Learning Initiative Working Paper. University of the Western Cape, South Africa; SEED Trust, South Africa. [www.globalhealthtrust.org/].

Loewenson, Rene. "Participation and Accountability in Health Systems: The Missing Factor in Equity?" Training and Research Support Center, Harare,

Zimbabwe. [Retrieved October 4, 2004, from www.equinetafrica.org/bibl/docs/partic&account.pdf].

Lyons, Maryinez. 1994. "The Power to Heal: African Medical Auxiliaries in Colonial Belgian Congo and Uganda." In Shula Marks and Dagmar Engels, eds., *Contesting Colonial Hegemony: State and Society in Africa and India, 1858 Until Independence*. London: British Academic Press.

Manderson, Lenore, Luzviminda Valencia, and Ben Thomas. 1992. "Bringing the People In: Community Participation and the Control of Tropical Disease." Resource Paper for Social and Economic Research in Tropical Disease 1. United Nations Development Programme/World Bank/World Health Organization Special Program for Research and Training in Tropical Diseases.

Mbele-Mbong, Lisa. 2001. "Human Capacity Development: Sustaining Local Responses through the Long Term." In French Ministry of Foreign Affairs, *Improving Access to Care in Developing Countries: Lessons from Practice, Research, Resources, and Partnerships*. Report from the meeting "Advocating for Access to Care and Sharing Experiences," November 29–December 1, Paris. Geneva: Joint United Nations Programme on HIV/AIDS, World Health Organization, French Ministry of Foreign Affairs.

Melgaard, B., A. Creese, B. Aylward, J. M. Olive, C. Mahler, J. M. Okwo-Bele, and J. W. Lee. 1998. "Disease Eradication and Health Systems Development." *Bulletin of the World Health Organization* 76 (Suppl. 2): 26–31.

Mumtaz, Zubia, Sarah Salway, Muneeba Waseem, and Nighat Umer. 2003. "Gender-Based Barriers to Primary Health Care Provision in Pakistan: The Experience of Female Providers." *Health Policy and Planning* 18 (3): 261–69.

Nakyanzi T. 1999. "Promoting Collaboration." *AIDS Action* 46:4.

PAHO (Pan American Health Organization). 2002. *Profile of the Health Services System of Costa Rica*. Washington, D.C.

Preker, Alexander S., Guy Carrin, David Dor, Melitta Jakab, William Hsiao, and Dyna Arhin-Tenkorang. 2002. "Effectiveness of Community Health Financing in Meeting the Cost of Illness." *Bulletin of the World Health Organization* 80 (2): 143–50.

Pretorius, Engela. 1999. "Traditional Healers." In Nicholas Crisp, ed., *South African Health Review 1999*. Durban: Health Systems Trust. [www.hst.org.za/sahr].

Ramirez-Valles, J. 1998. "Promoting Health, Promoting Women: The Construction of Female and Professional Identities in the Discourse of Community Health Workers." *Social Science and Medicine* 47 (11): 1749–62.

Reid, Steven, and Daphney Conco. 1999. "Monitoring the Implementation of Community Service." In Nicholas

Crisp, ed., *South African Health Review 1999*. Durban: Health Systems Trust. [www.hst.org.za/sahr].

Roemer, Milton I. 1991. *National Health Systems of the World: Volume I: The Countries*. Oxford: Oxford University Press.

———. 1993. *National Health Systems of the World: Volume II: The Issues*. Oxford: Oxford University Press.

Rohde, J. E., and H. Viswanathan. 1995. *The Rural Private Practitioner*. New Delhi: Oxford University Press.

Saengtienchai, C., and J. Knodel. 2001. Parents *Providing Care to Adult Sons and Daughters with HIV/AIDS in Thailand*. UNAIDS Best Practice Collection. Joint United Nations Programme on HIV/AIDS. [Retrieved October 4, 2004, from http://aidseld.psc.isr.umich.edu/sons_daughters.pdf].

Sanders, David. 1992. "The State and Democratization in Primary Health Care: Community Participation and the Village Health Worker Program in Zimbabwe." In S. Frankel, ed., *The Community Health Worker: Effective Programs for Developing Countries*. Oxford: Oxford University Press.

Troskie, T. R. 1997. "The Importance of Traditional Midwives in the Delivery of Health Care in the Republic of South Africa." *Curationis* 20 (1): 15–20.

Tshabalala-Msimang, Manto. 2004. "Substantial Allowances Ready to Roll for Health Professionals." Media Release. Government of South Africa, Department of Health, Pretoria.

UNDP (United Nations Development Programme). 1995. *Human Development Report 1995: Gender and Human Development*. New York: Oxford University Press.

van Rensburg, Dingie, and Nicolaas van Rensburg. 1999. "Distribution of Human Resources." In Nicholas Crisp, ed., *South African Health Review 1999*. Durban: Health Systems Trust. [www.hst.org.za/sahr].

Visschedijk, J., and P. Feenstra. 2003. *ILEP Technical Guide: Facilitating the Integration Process: A Guide to the Integration of Leprosy Services within the General Health System*. London: International Federation of Anti-Leprosy Associations.

Visschedijk, J., A. Engelhard, M. A. de Faria Grossi, and P. Feenstra. 2003. "Leprosy Control Strategies and the Integration of Health Services: An International Perspective." *Cadernos Saúde Pública* 19 (6): 1567–81. [Retrieved October 4, 2004, from www.scielosp.org/].

Walker, Damian, and Stephen Jan. 2004. "The Cost-Effectiveness of Community Health Workers: A Review of the Literature and Methodological Critique." Joint Learning Initiative Working Paper. University of Warwick, United Kingdom and London School of Hygiene and Tropical Medicine. [www.globalhealthtrust.org/].

Walt, G. 1990. *Community Health Workers in National Health Programmes: Just Another Pair of Hands?* London: Open University Press.

W.K. Kellogg Foundation. Undated. "UNI: Community Partnerships for Health Professions Education." [Retrieved October 4, 2004, from www.wkkf.org/pubs/Pub3358.pdf].

WHO (World Health Organization). 1987. "Community Health Workers: Pillars for Health for All." Report of the Interregional Conference, December 1–5, 1986, Yaoundé, Cameroon.

———. 1989. "Strengthening the Performance of Community Health Workers in Primary Health Care." Report of a WHO Study Group. WHO Technical Report Series 780. Geneva.

———. 2000. *World Health Report 2000: Health Systems: Improving Performance*. Geneva.

———. 2003. "The Costa Rican Health System: Low Cost, High Value." *Bulletin of the World Health Organization* 81 (8): 626–27.

———. 2004. *Gender and the Global Health Workforce: Information from 3 Key Sources*. Geneva.

WHO Regional Office for South-East Asia. 1996. "Role of Health Volunteers in Strengthening Community Action for Health." Report of an Inter-Country Consultation, February 20–24, 1995, Yangon.

Wibulpolprasert, Suwit, and Paichit Pengpaibon. 2003. "Integrated Strategies to Tackle the Inequitable Distribution of Doctors in Thailand: Four Decades of Experience." *Human Resources for Health* 1 (12).

Wilkinson D., L. Gcabashe, and M. Lurie. 1999. "Traditional Healers as Tuberculosis Treatment Supervisors: Precedent and Potential." *International Journal of Tuberculosis and Lung Disease* 3 (9): 838–42.

World Bank. 2004. *World Development Report 2004: Making Services Work for Poor People*. New York: Oxford University Press.

Wyss, Kaspar. 2004. "Human Resources for Health Development for Scaling-up Anti-Retroviral Treatment in Tanzania." World Health Organization, Department of Human Resources for Health, Geneva.

Country leadership

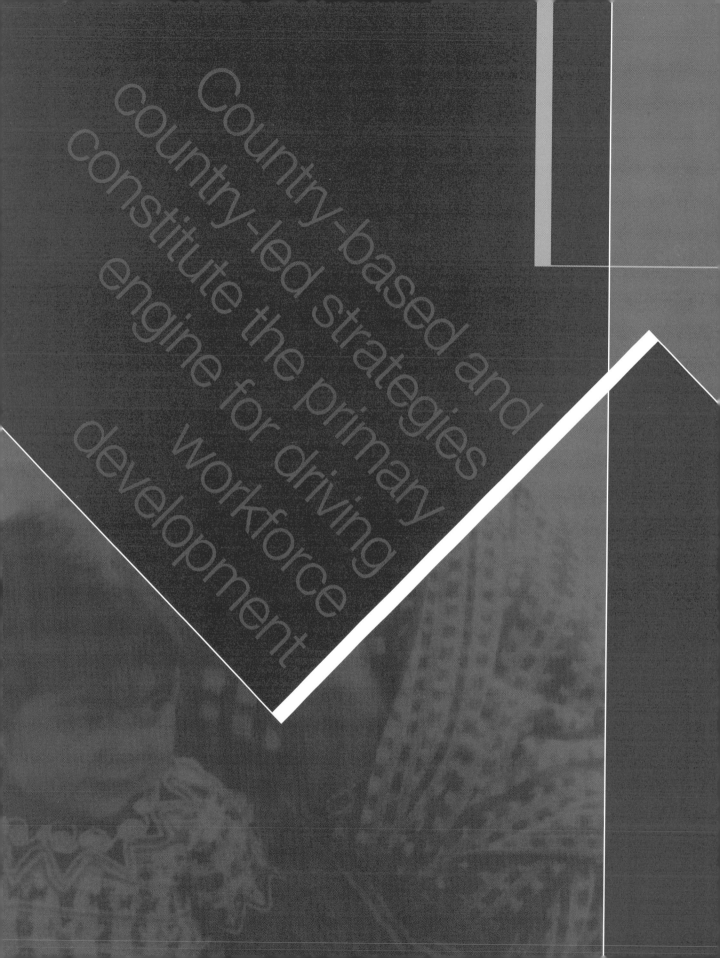

Country-based and
country-led strategies
constitute the primary
engine for driving
workforce
development

CHAPTER three

Country Leadership

Country-based and country-led strategies constitute the primary engine for driving workforce development. Why? Because the principal lever for strategic action is national. While frontline service delivery takes place in communities, workers at the local level require national government support in training, supplies, and financing. Although international knowledge and tools are important, it is at the country level that they are used and implemented. Most important, the effectiveness of workforce strategies depends on strategic planning and management being uniquely shaped to diverse national contexts. Although lessons may be shared across borders, a "cookie-cutter" approach to the workforce simply does not work.

Country strategies have five key dimensions:

- Engaging leaders and stakeholders
- Planning human investments
- Managing for performance
- Developing enabling policies
- Learning for improvement

This five-dimensional approach can infuse freshness into established policies and practices. It can also pull together and energize fragmented efforts (figure 3.1). Because workforce development is a "political-technical" process, the approach explicitly recognizes that national leaders and stakeholders are essential. It adopts a worker-centered perspective for planning and management, considering upstream education as crucial for building the downstream human infrastructure of health systems. It also adopts a systemic view of the health workforce, harmonizing health and education systems and the public and private sectors.

National experiences show that adopting such a strategic approach to workforce development

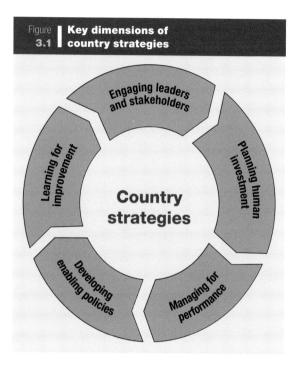

Figure 3.1 | **Key dimensions of country strategies**

Engaging leaders and stakeholders

Planning human investment

Learning for improvement

Country strategies

Developing enabling policies

Managing for performance

These payoffs to a strategic approach to workforce development are available to all countries, from those that face severe worker shortages to those with high, even excessive, worker density. Wealthy countries with high worker density, for example, have mature health and educational systems, usually staffed by well-established professional cadres. Their national priority is to contain costs, improve quality, and expand coverage to the disadvantaged. Such countries may concentrate on planning investments in education and managing health systems for performance with the luxury of a longer term horizon. Professional associations play the dual role of setting quality standards and ethical behavior while protecting professional interests.

Much harder pressed are countries with low worker densities and severe shortages. Many are poor, and many suffer from an unprecedented HIV/AIDS-related health crisis. Confronting medical emergencies, they have to overcome severe worker shortages, weak retention practices, and poor synchronization of such inputs as drugs and supplies. Many of them also have to coordinate massive infusions of donor funds. Their immediate priority is to stem the loss of workers due to negative work environments, the out-migration of highly skilled professionals, and AIDS-related deaths—while investing wisely for the immediate and long terms.

Engaging leaders and stakeholders

Workforce development is mistakenly perceived as either personnel administration or impossibly complicated. Purely technical approaches have often proven frustratingly ineffectual. Getting "the process right" is critical for success.

Workforce development should be seen as a political-technical process, shaped by history,

can generate large health payoffs, both improving the performance of the national health system and generating better health results. Thailand, over four decades, delivered services to remote rural populations by developing an innovative package of incentives for health workers.[1] Young doctors and nurses, qualifying for hardship and nonpractice allowances, could earn nearly as much as the most senior official. Brazil, supported by a series of national consultations with stakeholders, developed multiskilled "family health teams" to extend basic services to poor and disadvantaged communities.[2] Iran, over two decades, closed its rural-urban child mortality gap with a workforce strategy that linked paid "behvarze" workers and female community volunteers to "rural health houses," which were dispersed equitably throughout the countryside.[3]

**❝❝ Moving stakeholders to a consensus
requires political commitment
and national leadership**

bureaucratic procedures, labor markets, and political accommodations of diverse interests. It requires leadership and political negotiations to develop consensus. There are few cases of successful health sector reform without at least the acquiescence of workers and their associations. As a service industry, the health sector cannot perform without the support, participation, and enthusiasm of its workers, keeping in mind that worker interests are multidimensional, ranging from financial self-interest to heroic social dedication.

Government stakeholders go beyond the ministry of health to include ministries of finance, education, planning, labor, and the civil service. All these sectors must cooperate to generate an enabling environment for health. Stakeholders also go beyond governmental bodies to include academic institutions, private clinics and hospitals, health industries, nongovernmental organizations, and consumer groups. And through their professional associations and worker unions, workers are key stakeholders. Ignoring them is a recipe for failure, for some worker associations—of doctors, for example—can be at times even more powerful than politicians.[4]

In many low-income countries, stakeholders also include the decisionmakers for key international programs, agencies, and development partners— because of the financial and technical resources they invest. Harmonizing external inputs into country decisionmaking is an important element of the national political-technical process.

Stakeholders must strive to develop a consensus on national health goals, test and implement solutions, and make adjustments based on feedback from monitoring. It must be explicitly recognized that health priorities may vary among

the relevant stakeholders in any country. Some may set priorities for specific problems, such as polio, tuberculosis, or cardiovascular disease. Some may see HIV/AIDS as a national medical emergency. Others may focus on health system development, perhaps access to improved primary health care. Still others may push to reduce child and maternal mortality—to reach the Millennium Development Goals. And for workers or professional associations, salary levels, professional status, and working conditions may be at the forefront of the agenda.

All these goals are legitimate, but each has different implications for workforce priorities. In every country, priority setting must be accommodated among diverse stakeholders. In some intractable situations, where a consensus among stakeholders cannot be achieved immediately, pilot projects and demonstration sites can be set up for new initiatives—evaluating changes, soliciting feedback, and engaging opinion leaders in an ongoing dialogue on the health workforce.

Moving stakeholders to a consensus requires political commitment and national leadership. The health workforce, customarily considered a backwater field, has generally been neglected. Because of long investment-to-yield times, the political payoffs are not immediate. Leadership is thus crucial to strengthen national ownership of workforce strategies. An open consultative process can help focus on shared goals, navigating interest groups toward more effective workforce development. A prominent national champion can come from within or outside of government—to bring stakeholders together and raise the profile of health workers.

Sound organizational arrangements are needed to engage key stakeholders and firmly root the

> **❝ The health workforce supply should be adapted to constantly changing demand, and the health system should be adapted to a constantly changing workforce supply**

process in country action. To plan and set policies, Kenya established an intersectoral collaboration committee based in the president's office. Tanzania established a working group for human resources in the ministry of health and assigned tasks to its public service commission. At regular intervals, Brazil brings together stakeholders in "Conferencias Nacionais de Saude," in which health worker issues have regularly been high on the agenda.[5] Commonwealth countries, following British tradition, have regularly used "commissions of enquiry" to grapple with workforce issues. National processes can also link to donor mechanisms—such as the Heavily Indebted Poor Country Initiative, Millennium Development Goals, poverty reduction strategies, sector-wide approaches, and national AIDS coordination mechanisms.

But there are no shortcuts. Stakeholders are critical to every aspect of strategy development and execution. Workers are active agents, not passive commodities. They are not fungible in the way money can be. Nor are they easily moved, the way drugs and supplies can be. Experience has repeatedly shown that workers can be a powerful lever—or obstacle—in changing health systems (box 3.1).

Planning human investments

All countries should have updated plans for workforce development to guide investments in education and health for building the human infrastructure of future health systems. But such plans often do not exist or, if they do, are not implemented.

Planning is an exercise in investing financial, human, and institutional resources for the future. "Plan long, act short, and update often" could well be a guiding principle for health workforce planning, which must adopt long, medium, and short term

horizons.[6] All countries should maintain longer term planning horizons because advanced professional competencies require more than a decade of planned investments, and good education requires strong and stable institutions. These investments can generate high and sustained human yields but only after a long period of gestation to maturity. For most countries the medium term is more reliably predicted, and thus the linkages between investment and return are more concrete. For some countries, especially those facing a dire health situation, planning must tackle the immediate workforce crisis.

Health systems all have many interactive and interdependent parts. They consist of free agents who act in not fully controllable ways, and whose actions can change the playing field for others. Workforce development cannot be done separately from health system development planning or from broader societal developments—in economics, education, politics, markets, and cultural change.

How can planning create a flexible health workforce for rapidly changing health systems? The first requirement is to ensure that accurate information is collected on the size, skills, and distribution of the workforce (for planning methods, see box 4.5). Current workforce data often do not include annual supply or loss rates, private sector characteristics, or staff productivity. And planning tools may not be suitable in low-income countries. Computer modeling can provide valuable simulations for planners—to allow them to explore alternatives and involve stakeholders in making choices. Marginal budgeting for bottlenecks is one example, usefully applied in several African countries. But simulations provide possibilities rather than answers. Even with simulations, planners still have to choose among possible health worker

Box
3.1 | **Workers on strike**

3

COUNTRY LEADERSHIP

Imagine working for months at a time without receiving a paycheck or the other allowances you are entitled to. Imagine working for two years without a formal contract. Imagine your salary being frozen while the conditions you work in are deteriorating. These are the difficulties facing health care workers around the world. And these are some of the reasons why workers go on strike.

At any point in time, there are literally a handful of ongoing health worker strikes paralyzing health systems around the world. An internet search of news sources found more than 40 industrial actions by doctors, nurses, and other health care providers in the six months from September 2003 to February 2004. The actions ranged from strikes lasting several months to slowdowns, sit-ins, and other protests—all paralyzing or hurting health service provision. No part of the world is immune. The most common grievance cited by workers was low pay. Other common reasons included demands for better working conditions and the provision of housing allowances, protests over government plans for the privatization of the health sector and medical education, and demands for better on-the-job protection from contagious diseases.

Some examples:

Côte d'Ivoire—Nurses in Côte d'Ivoire's government-run hospitals and health centers began an indefinite strike to demand protection from contagious diseases following the death of six nurses from infections contracted from their patients.

Ecuador—After the government announced that it was freezing salaries of 100,000 state employees for two years, health workers, including medics and paramedics, went on an indefinite strike, closing down 202 hospitals and health centers.

Italy—Tens of thousands of Italian doctors and other public sector health workers staged a one-day strike over delayed contract renewals and low government expenditures. It was the first occasion on which all 42 trade unions representing health workers had gone on strike simultaneously.

Mali—The National Union of Malian Workers, including the National Union of Health Workers, launched a two-day strike over the government's delay in revising the salary scale and the great wage disparity between contractual workers and their integrated counterparts in the public service.

Nigeria—Medical doctors in the Federal Medical Centre,

Bayelsa State, embarked on an indefinite industrial action because they were paid only 82 percent of their December 2003 and January 2004 salaries.

Peru—The Peruvian Physicians' Federation staged a 25-day strike demanding wage increases that ended in mid-December, the fourth instance of industrial action by health workers in the country since October.

Sri Lanka—75,000 health workers, including laborers, attendants and clerks, went on a six-day strike in state hospitals, demanding higher wages. Health services were severely affected as government deployed the armed forces to help maintain hospital care.

Turkey—Health workers across the country went on strike to protest low salaries and poor working conditions. The Turkish Doctors' Union organized protests to demand an increase in the percentage of the national budget allotted to health care and to demand better working conditions.

Zambia—Scores of junior doctors, nurses and support staff went on an indefinite strike at Zambia's largest hospital, the University Teaching Hospital in Lusaka, over unpaid housing allowances.

Source: Africa News 2003a, 2004b; Deutsche Presse-Agentur 2003a, 2003b; *Financial Times* 2004; Panafrican News Agency 2003a, 2003b; Scavino 2003; *Turkish Daily News* 2003.

> **"** **Planning should be an ongoing process of goal setting, information gathering, analysis, evaluation, and adaptation**

scenarios and use the results to influence the production and deployment of health workers.

Countries are using more sophisticated methods to plan for their health workers. Most approaches now have both a normative and empirical component and analyze the many factors that influence the health workforce, looking at labor market forces, economic development, education, and attrition rates.[7] And most go beyond just counting numbers, types, or locations to include management: of roles, functions, production, deployment, recruitment, retention, and remuneration.

Agility, adaptability, and flexibility can be supported by analyses of needs and gaps.[8] Coping with complexity means not only meeting projected workforce gaps but also assessing job shifts over time, changing worker expectations, and shifting labor markets—anticipating and accommodating changes in health systems. Moving beyond simple planning-to-action relationships, incentives, regulations, certification, and information can be used to shape positive workforce developments. The key message in planning is adaptability. The health workforce supply should be adapted to constantly changing demand, and the health system should be adapted to a constantly changing workforce supply. Planning must also navigate the private labor markets imbedded in health service markets.

In the real world, the demand and supply of health services are not well matched to national health needs.[9] The mismatch is due to both market failures and public system failures. Rather than meeting genuine national health needs, health service supply and demand reflect the "inverse care law"—that services are distributed inversely to needs. In other words, those whose need for services is greatest are often located where there is the least access.[10]

Workforce strategies should thus align the supply and demand for workers to the provision of services. The demand for services comes from clients, but the effective demand for workers comes from employer organizations that have the institutions and resources to create job opportunities. A major challenge to planning is to encourage both public and private sector developments to meet national health needs. Health workers, like all workers, operate through labor markets that are mostly local and national but increasingly international—driving workers across public-private sectors and geographic regions.

Planning must also extend beyond the health sector. Probably the most limiting aspect of current planning methods is their confinement to ministries of health. Yet other sectors powerfully influence the workforce environment. Planning should ensure supportive policies in education, finance, and the civil service. Especially relevant are the growth and development of appropriate educational capacity that ensures equitable access for both men and women. Budget allocations are obviously key parameters in determining realistic options for workforce development. Most important, however, is that planning not be limited to the production of a national planning document. It should be an ongoing process of goal setting, information gathering, analysis, evaluation, and adaptation.

Managing for performance

Strategic management should aim to achieve positive health outcomes from a better performing health system—and from more productive health workers. One way to consider performance and productivity is through the goals of equitable access, efficiency and effectiveness, and quality and responsiveness (figure 3.2).[11] These performance

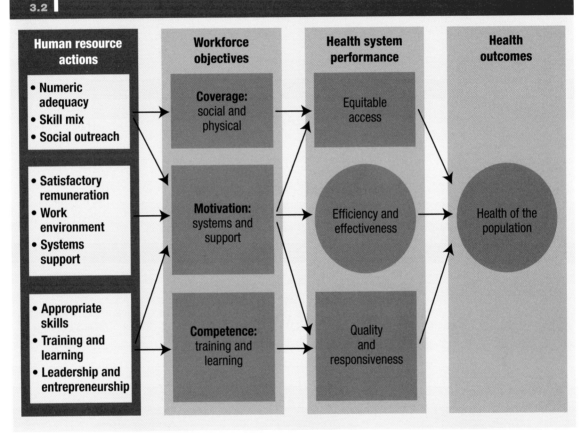

Figure 3.2 | Managing for performance

Human resource actions	Workforce objectives	Health system performance	Health outcomes
• Numeric adequacy • Skill mix • Social outreach	Coverage: social and physical	Equitable access	
• Satisfactory remuneration • Work environment • Systems support	Motivation: systems and support	Efficiency and effectiveness	Health of the population
• Appropriate skills • Training and learning • Leadership and entrepreneurship	Competence: training and learning	Quality and responsiveness	

parameters, in turn, are shaped by three core workforce objectives—coverage, motivation, and competence, each of them affected by workforce strategies. Coverage depends on numerically sufficient and appropriately skilled workers well distributed for physical and social access. Motivation is promoted by satisfactory remuneration, a positive work environment, and systems that support the worker. Competence requires education with an appropriate orientation and curriculum, continuing learning, and fostering innovation and leadership.

The framework may appear simple and linear, but its elements are interactive and can be complex. Coverage is determined not simply by the number of workers but by their skill mix, their geographic placement, the resources and support at their disposal, and their social compatibility with clients. Many countries that have large numbers of workers are still unable to generate full coverage of their populace because of skill misfits or geographic maldistributions. Similarly, a deficiency in health workers may signal a need for

> **National strategies should expand coverage by ensuring numeric adequacy, developing appropriate worker mixes, and pushing for rural and social outreach**

a stronger educational infrastructure for training doctors and nurses—or a sign of inappropriate production targets that should instead provide for briefer training of more auxiliary workers.

Coverage

All countries, rich and poor, suffer from the physical and social inaccessibility of services, with deficiencies relating to both overall coverage and the inability to reach poor or marginal populations. Deficient coverage has several elements: absolute numeric insufficiency, inappropriate skill mixes, geographic maldistributions, and the social distance between workers and clients. The gaps affect almost all health efforts, ranging from primary care to tuberculosis control and polio eradication.

National shortages are extreme examples of a global worker shortage. The total global deficit of doctors, nurses, and midwives, assuming that all countries should attain an average worker density of 2.5 per 1,000 population, would be about 4 million (chapter 1).

Numeric deficiency is related to worker skill mixes that hinder the delegation of tasks to less expensive auxiliaries. This is illustrated in the nurse-to-doctor ratio. High ratios of nurses to doctors allow for efficiency gains through delegation of key tasks from fewer doctors to more numerous nurses. Yet the potential for delegation varies enormously. Each doctor in Thailand and in countries in the Commonwealth of Independent States has 5 to 10 nurses, but in Brazil and Colombia there is only one nurse for every three doctors.[12]

Geographic maldistributions are a clear example of market failure.[13] Labor markets will not attract highly skilled workers to poor and remote regions.

And physicians posted in rural areas are typically younger, less experienced, and less likely to remain in their posts over the long term. Rural worker neglect and urban worker concentration are common in all countries. Data from Ghana, Nicaragua, Mexico, and Bangladesh document this urban bias.[14] Richer countries have the same problems as poorer countries. In Canada, for instance, there are significant variations in the average physician to population ratio between provinces.[15] Even exporting countries like the Philippines, India, and Egypt have problems. While they purposefully produce workers for export, they simultaneously have domestic coverage gaps in rural and marginal regions.

Social barriers can also compromise access to care. Worker attributes and capabilities—such as language, gender, ethnicity, religion, and class—can ease or block provider-client relationships. In most societies, the gender composition of the workforce influences access to women's health and reproductive services.

National strategies should aim to expand coverage by ensuring numeric adequacy, developing appropriate worker mixes, and pushing for rural and social outreach.

Ensuring numeric adequacy. Ensuring numeric adequacy is a huge challenge for severe deficit countries, especially in sub-Saharan Africa. Accepting a minimum baseline of 2.5 workers per 1,000 population, sub-Saharan countries would immediately require an additional 1 million doctors, nurses, and midwives. Ethiopia would require an additional 150,000 workers, about the number of health workers in Belgium.[16] To deliver priority MDG interventions, Tanzania would have to triple

**" The stock of workers can also be expanded through
massive investment and acceleration in medical education
for professionals and in training for auxiliary health workers**

and Chad to quadruple their worker numbers by 2015. Botswana—well-endowed with health workers by African standards—would require a doubling of nurses, a tripling of physicians, and a quintupling of pharmacists to achieve its national goal of freely accessible antiretroviral treatment for all eligible HIV-positive citizens.[17]

Numeric adequacy is not simply a matter of numbers. It is closely linked to work environments. As long as existing workers are not retained or productive, adding more will not be effective. There are cases, however, where massive shortages must be urgently corrected. Immediate and wholesale expansion of the health workforce in countries facing severe shortages of workers could, in theory, be accomplished by hiring trained health workers now unemployed or employed in other sectors, or by importing workers, including the repatriation of workers abroad. Several thousand health workers are currently unemployed in countries facing shortages, including South Africa and Kenya.[18] Targeted campaigns to recruit these workers back into the health sector could yield huge and immediate numeric gains for the health workforce in these countries. Importing workers could also have a rapid impact. To gain a sense of the magnitude of worker movement required, meeting sub-Saharan Africa's gap of 1 million workers could be accomplished by importing 10 percent of the 11 million OECD doctors, nurses, and midwives. This is clearly unrealistic as global flows of health workers are moving instead the other way, with workers from sub-Saharan Africa and other developing regions going to OECD countries.

The stock of workers can also be expanded through massive investment and acceleration in medical education for professionals and in training

for auxiliary health workers. Clearly the competencies that could be developed among newly trained workers are a tradeoff against the time and investments required. It would be impossible, for example, to double doctor or nursing numbers within a decade. A more appropriate strategy would focus on building up cadres of briefly trained and well-supported auxiliary workers who can perform core basic functions. It would be very difficult for the health sector to achieve this massive expansion without an alliance with the education sector. And it will be essential to ensure that new health workers are not recruited at the expense of other essential sectors, such as education and agricultural extension. (A later section explores complementary actions to enhance worker retention, reduce attrition, and stem out-migration.)

Developing an appropriate worker mix. In many countries there is no possibility of meeting the population's health needs with the existing mix of worker types, skills, and training. The massive gap calls for different approaches.

High and low-income countries alike are using or considering "new" health workers, such as multiskilled generic care assistants, nurse practitioners, nurse anesthetists, and doctors' assistants. The new worker is often a current occupation or grade, with additional skills or an expanded role. Many of these amended roles fall into one of four categories:[19]

- Multiskilled or extended roles for traditional support workers, such as workers with catering, patient transport, cleaning, and clerical duties.
- Cross-training for care assistants and auxiliaries, such as community health agents in Brazil's family health program.[20]

" Greater gender equity in the workforce will generally enhance women's recruitment and retention in the health workforce

- Extended roles for current health care professionals, such as nurse practitioners.
- New technician roles, as for surgery and anesthesiology in such countries as Mozambique.[21]

Mobilizing auxiliary cadres of health workers has been effective in diverse countries. Clinical officers, medical assistants, and clinical outreach nurses have become the backbone of health service delivery in many sub-Saharan countries. Paramedical staff now manage urgent surgical interventions in Malawi and Tanzania.[22] Botswana has developed nurse practitioners and para-pharmacists.[23] Mozambique and Ethiopia have trained field surgeons and clinical officers.[24] And Ghana has rural midwives with life-saving skills for maternity cases.[25] In revamping its workforce, Iran developed tens of thousands of behvarzes and female volunteers. Brazil has developed a national network of "community health agents." These workers and many others like them have repeatedly demonstrated that they can offer simple preventive and curative services to underserved populations.

The delegation of a controlled set of tasks to auxiliary workers, though an important opportunity for improving coverage, also faces several obstacles. National leadership may not seize the opportunity to increase auxiliary development, or ministry planners may be confined within a doctor-nurse paradigm for service delivery. There are also legacies of colonialism that resist "second class" worker categories.[26] Most common, professional associations oppose and resist the delegation of tasks to other cadres of workers.[27] Resistance to delegation may be found not only among elite doctors but other skilled workers like laboratory technicians. This underscores the

importance of engaging these groups as stakeholders to make national workforce strategies politically viable.

Promoting rural and social outreach. No country has fully corrected its geographic imbalances. Various incentives and regulations have had mixed success. Some of these approaches include providing educational scholarships in return for taking on rural or hardship posts after graduation, assuring access to equipment and supplies, providing communications to maintain contact with peers and supervisors, increasing security measures to attract female providers, offering opportunities to upgrade competencies, granting future access to specialized training, and accelerating promotion and career development paths. Indonesia and Thailand hold specialist training slots for workers who have completed rural service to improve rural access to workers.[28] South Africa and Malawi have used bonding or compulsory service regulations to shift the geographic distribution in countries, though they have been difficult to monitor and enforce.[29]

Far more effective, but also far more demanding of long-term planning and investment, are appropriate educational policies upstream. Locating training institutions in marginal regions rather than national capitals helps to bias workers toward disadvantaged regions. Recruiting and selecting students from rural communities improves the odds that graduates will be willing to serve in rural placements. As Brazil, Indonesia, and Thailand show, graduates are much more likely to return to their home communities if their education was selected or supported by the local community.

Recruiting students from diverse backgrounds—by gender, language, age, ethnicity, and cultural tradition—can also help in the social alignment of

> **❝ Our personal safety is not guaranteed. Patients are harassing us, and shouting at us. They have guns and you are not expected to retaliate, to say anything to them, because it is said they are right.**
>
> —*Primary health care nurse, South Africa*[30]

workers with their patients. Greater gender equity in the workforce will generally enhance women's recruitment and retention in the health workforce. But more investments will need to be made to ensure that, despite the family considerations of female workers, there are incentives and opportunities for them to serve in remote regions.

Motivation

Motivation, undoubtedly the most critical worker attribute driving performance, is generated by a complex combination of factors including: personal values, professional ethics, remuneration, the work environment, and the support of the health system. While skills and competencies usually receive more attention, these are of little worth without worker motivation. Money, drugs, and supplies are also wasted if a worker is not motivated. Health, after all, is a "human service." And for a service system to perform well, workers have to want to serve their clients.

The most common worker grievance is, not surprisingly, unsatisfactory compensation. Wages may not be sufficient for personal and family requirements. Salaries may not be adjusted for cycles of inflation. And salaries may not be paid on time. In many countries, civil service wages have fallen dramatically in recent years. In Tanzania a civil servant's wage in 1998 was only 70 percent of that in 1969. Wage freezes have shifted resources to allowances and nonfinancial incentives. With wages in Jordan frozen since 1988, allowances now make up 70 percent of the base salary. Allowances in Indonesia, meanwhile, are more than 90 percent of total compensation. Low wages in the public sector can drive workers out of the country or encourage dual practices, with public

servants providing private services.[31] Dual practices can set off a conflict of interest as workers devote less time and attention to public service, and jostle for assignments in more lucrative urban centers. At its worst, inadequate worker compensation can spawn predatory worker behavior—marketing and selling of drugs, or demanding illegal payments for services.

Poor working conditions and management cultures also reduce worker motivation. The complaints of health workers are common to other sectors as well: heavy workloads, burn out, too many administrative duties, isolation from colleagues, insufficient team work, and occupational hazards. The lack of recognition, the discouragement of new ideas, and the lack of career opportunities are also all demotivating, often leading to absenteeism (box 3.2).

Management structures often lack transparent policies and good communication practices. And too often workers feel as though their managers care very little about their concerns and well-being. A study in Burkina Faso found that more than half of health workers were dissatisfied with their working conditions due to factors ranging from poor management systems to inadequate resources and support to unfair regulations.[32] Ombudsmen for dispute resolution are very rare. Many of these problems have been even more pronounced as public sector wage freezes have taken effect, workforces have been downsized, and workplaces have become even more fraught with resentment and misunderstanding.

No matter how hard-working and dedicated workers are, they know that their efforts will be futile without medicines or technology. The decay of infrastructure and the absence of drugs and supplies are not only discouraging—they are also limiting. Remote clinics can wait months to

❝❝ **They pretend to pay us,
and we pretend to work.**

—*Participant at JLI Consultation*

Box 3.2 | Ghosts and absentee workers

Some health systems are plagued by "ghost" and "absent" workers. Ghost workers are nonexistent, listed in the payroll, and paid, a clear sign of corruption. Absenteeism can be a significant barrier to the effective provision of health services. The problem is twofold. Vacancy rates describe unfilled posts, particularly in rural areas where providers are unwilling to go. Absentee rates characterize filled posts with absent providers. While a very large percentage of public spending on health goes toward salaries—reaching 80–90 percent—this money is wasted if many workers are not on the job. Correcting these corrupt practices can sometimes be dangerous work.

A recent study in which unannounced visits were made to 150 health facilities in Bangladesh found very high absentee and vacancy rates. The average number of vacancies for all types of health workers was 26 percent—and vacancy rates, or unfilled posts, were generally even higher in poorer parts of the country. Although there was great variation in absentee rates across types of workers, rates were particularly high for doctors, with an average absentee rate of over 40 percent. At smaller subcenters, the rate climbed to over 70 percent.

Absenteeism has been documented in countries around the world. The absence of health care providers, particularly of doctors, has been shown to adversely affect the number of patients visiting a health facility as well as the quality of services. These effects are particularly pronounced for people living in rural areas, where access to health services is already a serious issue. Yet there have been few systematic efforts to fully understand and correct widespread health worker absenteeism—perhaps because of the dangers in revealing it. Effective national plans to combat it must combine better understanding of the size of the problem with policy interventions that see health care providers as active decisionmakers.

Source: Chaudhury and Hammer 2003.

---

receive supplies during rainy seasons. In 2004 all qualified health workers in the remote Melekoza district in southern Ethiopia vacated their posts because of a lack of supplies, leaving 100,000 people in the care of a single sanitarian with only two years of post-secondary training.[33]

Violence, threats, and abuse also impair worker motivation. It is estimated that almost 25 percent of all workplace violence occurs in the health sector—and that more than half of healthcare workers globally are estimated to have been affected by workplace violence.[34] Many times, threats to worker safety are beyond the control of the health sector. Extension workers often travel alone in remote areas or are compelled to travel at unsafe hours or in unsafe neighborhoods. Health facilities also can house hostile work environments.

Studies from Portugal and South Africa suggest that female health workers are especially likely to be the targets of physical abuse and sexual harassment.[35] South African nurses, most of them women, are three times more likely than other occupational groups to experience violence in the workplace.[36] Potential exposure to HIV/AIDS while on the job is another safety concern. And despite the risk of infection, many health workers do not or cannot take the precautions to protect themselves.

National approaches to enhance motivation should aim at satisfactory remuneration, a positive work environment, and synchronized support systems.

Achieving satisfactory remuneration. Worker compensation consists of wages, benefits, and allowances, and can be structured as salaries, fee-for-service opportunities, or capitation payments. Workers may never be entirely satisfied with their salaries, but in many countries the real wages of workers have fallen over recent years due to inflation and civil service and health sector reform. To improve worker motivation, remuneration should be continually reassessed to fall in line with budgetary capacity (from both domestic and external sources) and the cost of living.

In 1993 Uganda introduced a program that provided all staff employed in health facilities with a lunch allowance that would supplement their salaries. The allowance amounted to 66,600 Ugandan shillings a month for medical workers and 44,000 a month for support staff, an effective increase in pay of nearly 30 percent.[37] The lunch allowance appears to have dampened worker unrest in the short run, though in the long term it must be part of a wider effort to promote better salaries, benefits, and work environments.

Over the last several decades, Thailand has also pursued initiatives to improve health worker remuneration. Among the financial incentives are special allowances for physicians, dentists, and pharmacists who work in remote district hospitals or who agree not to engage in private practice.[38] The system has been able thus far to resist unaffordable

upward adjustments, citing budget constraints and equitable treatment of all public workers.

There is growing interest in linking compensation to worker performance. Rwanda and Kenya are considering incentive payments tied to performance indicators. Some nongovernmental organizations have used performance-based payments with great success. In Bangladesh BRAC has built compensation incentives into its oral rehydration and tuberculosis programs. The monthly salaries of workers training mothers in oral rehydration therapy against diarrhea are based on how well mothers learn. In the directly observed treatment (DOTS) program against tuberculosis, patients are required to pay an upfront fee for treatment. Part of the fee is returned to the patient upon successful completion of treatment, but part is retained by the health worker as an incentive for patient compliance.[39] Performance-linked financial incentives can help imbue public service values, a sense of purpose, and social recognition.

Most low-income countries need to control the damaging effects of "dual practice."[40] In Kenya strict prohibition against public sector workers in private practice was ineffective, and policies were adjusted to allow clinical officers and nurses to practice privately. Openly acknowledging and discussing the conflict of interest was a key element in resolving the issue to the satisfaction of government, workers, and clients.

Numerous studies point to the importance of nonfinancial incentives to worker motivation. More tangible incentives include: opportunities for career advancement and continuing education, access to training, flexible work hours, good employment conditions, adequate vacation time, and access to child care. Less tangible are social recognition, community esteem, and fulfilling

❝ **Ensuring worker access to drugs, supplies, information, and a functioning infrastructure is crucial to motivation**

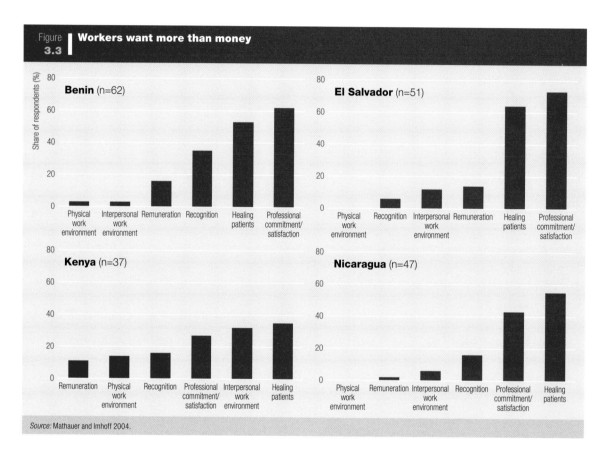

Figure 3.3 | **Workers want more than money**

Source: Mathauer and Imhoff 2004.

religious, spiritual, or philanthropic obligations. A recent survey of health workers in Kenya identified recognition, career advancement, team spirit, and promotion prospects among the nonfinancial factors that affected worker motivation (figure 3.3).[41] A similar range of nonfinancial incentives was reported by workers in the Indian state of Andhra Pradesh.[42] Gender sensitive arrangements—including flexible hours, part-time work, child care, training for career development—are especially important for female staff.[43]

Creating a positive work environment. Effective personnel management, structures, and strategies can foster a favorable work environment. Managers are called on to motivate workers, provide them with regular feedback, monitor workloads, and promote a culture of quality, where participation is valued above authoritarianism, where due process and not patronage is the norm, and where channels are open for communications between workers and managers. Good management practices include establishing norms and standards, supporting transparency and worker participation in decision-making, encouraging workers to solve problems

> **A positive work enviornment is at the core of the common observation that nongovernmental and faith-based organizations often retain a motivated staff with remuneration levels similar to, or even less than, those in the public sector**

and innovate, and promoting social and gender sensitivity. Professional associations, unions, faculties of medicine and nursing, and other educational institutions all have a responsibility to help workers pursue excellence, respect clients, and develop a culture of professionalism.

A positive work environment is at the core of the common observation that nongovernmental and faith-based organizations often retain a motivated staff with remuneration levels similar to, or even lower than, those in the public sector.[44] Especially important are their good management and systems that support worker initiative and innovation.[45] And family considerations and career prospects often are better addressed in nongovernmental organizations than in the public sector.

Synchronizing systems of support. Ensuring worker access to drugs, supplies, information, colleagues, and a functioning infrastructure for service provision is crucial to motivation. In a recent survey of health workers in Benin and Kenya, systems support—the materials and means necessary to do the work assigned—was the most often cited answer to the question of how to increase workers' spirit and willingness to perform.[46] Materials and means outranked salary, training, and recognition. Nongovernmental organizations often do better than the public sector in ensuring inputs for their workers, a key to a motivated and productive workforce. Where workforce development has been successful, as in Thailand, Brazil, and Iran, inputs have been synchronized.

An additional element of systems support is ensuring the physical safety of workers. Violence in the health workplace may be difficult to address, but

specific measures can communicate a message of "zero tolerance." Governments and other employers should make the reduction and prevention of workplace violence a key part of all human resource strategies and legislation. Workers should be encouraged to report all incidents of violence, no matter how minor, and ongoing support should be accessible to all workers affected. Health facility managers and governments should collect ongoing data on the incidence of workplace violence and its contributing factors—to develop effective local, regional, and national strategies to combat it.[47]

HIV/AIDS is increasing workloads, killing workers, and causing stress among care providers. In high-prevalence countries, protective equipment and safe practices should be developed to reduce worker risk. Ensuring adequate supplies of simple protective equipment (gloves, soap, and bleach), training workers in precautionary guidelines and protocols, and implementing post-exposure prophylaxis policies are all necessary to maintain a healthy workforce. Sustaining supplies will require effective logistic channels and adequate budget allocations at all levels of the health system. Given the key role of workers in advancing human security, health workers should be given free antiretroviral drug treatment—as in Zambia.[48]

Competence

The health education infrastructure is weak in the poorest countries. Of some 1,642 medical schools that together produce about 370,000 doctors each year, only 64 (4 percent) are situated in sub-Saharan Africa. In this subcontinent, 21 countries had one school and 6 countries had none.[49] Data on nursing schools are inadequate, and information on training for

" National strategies should aim at enhancing competencies by educating for appropriate skills, fostering leadership and entrepreneurship, and training for continual learning

Figure 3.4 | Huge regional disparities in medical schools and graduates

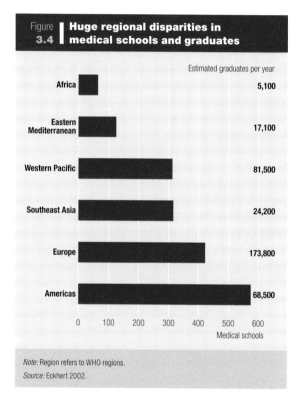

Estimated graduates per year

Region		Graduates
Africa		5,100
Eastern Mediterranean		17,100
Western Pacific		81,500
Southeast Asia		24,200
Europe		173,800
Americas		68,500

Medical schools

Note: Region refers to WHO regions.
Source: Eckhert 2002.

In most schools, the curriculum is misaligned with the country's health problems, and pedagogic methods are outdated, excluding practical problem-solving skills.[51] Production of health workers is based not on working competencies but on certification or traditional roles. Curricula and teaching typically follow the model of western medical standards and are often aligned to the goal of professional bodies—generating graduates who can enhance professional status, generate higher earnings, and increase the potential for out-migration to wealthier countries.

Major gaps are also found in continuing education. Short-term training is fragmented and episodic, suffering from a lack of coordination, follow-up, or integration into a worker's career plans. High-priority programs for HIV/AIDS, immunization, and child health often compete to secure trainees. Donors do not maintain records or inventories of their training activities, and few have conducted evaluations of their effectiveness.

Further diminishing the development of appropriate competencies in the health workforce is an environment that stifles learning and initiative rather than fostering leadership. In low and middle-income countries, there are few health leadership and management programs that encourage innovation and entrepreneurship.[52] Some programs emphasize individual skills, but few build team leadership. And the pedagogic effectiveness of leadership training and education has been difficult to assess.[53]

National strategies should aim at enhancing competencies by educating for appropriate skills, training for continual learning, and fostering leadership and entrepreneurship—all supported by a pipeline of learning investments in pre-service education and in-service training (figure 3.5).

other cadres is entirely absent. Educational capacity in public health is similarly constrained. A recent survey found that more than half of countries in Africa had no graduate training program in public health.[50] And many training institutions on the continent are only marginally equipped with teaching facilities, laboratories, journals, computers, and internet access.

The imbalance in the production of medical graduates is huge (figure 3.4). Europe produces 173,800 doctors a year, Africa only 5,100. One doctor is produced for every 5,000 people in Central and Eastern Europe and the Baltic States in comparison to one doctor for every 115,000 people in sub-Saharan Africa.

3

Figure 3.5 | **Investment pipeline of learning**

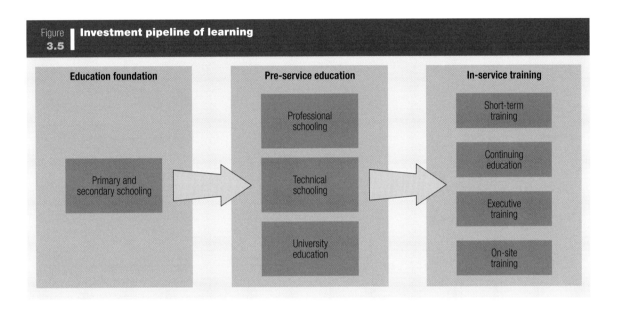

Educating for appropriate skills. Developing appropriate skills to meet health needs will require a dramatic expansion of educational production and major curricular reforms in most countries. National decisionmakers should dramatically expand pre-service educational capacity or shift the focus of production to new categories of auxiliary workers who can be produced more quickly and more cheaply. The volume of educational expansion required in severe deficit countries appears far beyond existing capabilities. Regional approaches to health professions education may be important. In some countries, the focus could be training auxiliary and community health workers—rather than expensive and time-consuming advanced professional training.

Numeric expansion must be coordinated with curricular reform. Experience from around the world suggests the importance of community-oriented, problem-based learning to future community-based

practice in both high and low-income settings. In addition to technical subjects, students should be exposed to social epidemiology and social and behavioral sciences. Field practice should supplement classroom study. Because graduates will have to adapt to new knowledge, techniques, and technologies throughout their careers, the curriculum should also teach how to maintain and sustain learning. The Towards Unity for Health Network is addressing these learning challenges by bringing together community-oriented medical schools to share curricula, courses, learning strategies, and educational developments (box 3.3).

Training for continuous learning. A strategic goal should be to propagate a "culture of active learning" for all cadres of health workers. Learning should be viewed as a life-long and career-long privilege and responsibility. Many types of training programs can encourage learning, such as continuing education, executive

Box 3.3 | **Networks for learning and health**

A worldwide association of NGOs, multilateral organizations, academic institutions, and many other groups and individuals, the **Network: Towards Unity for Health** is improving the relevance, performance, and accessibility of health services to address the needs of individuals and communities. In Brazil the Network forged a partnership between a women's collective, a local university, and a primary care clinic to have community workers survey homes and determine priority health needs. In Malaysia it was involved in designing a community-based curriculum for an interdisciplinary team of health professionals. A variety of networking events, consultations, conferences, and publications encourage mutual assistance and support among all stakeholders and members in the Network.

At the heart of another network is the **Virtual Campus for Public Health.** Launched in 2003 by the Pan American Health Organization in association with 14 academic institutions from the Americas and Spain, it offers distance learning courses for health personnel. Directed toward leaders and decisionmaking professionals in public health, public health professors, and public health professionals, the virtual courses, offered in English, Spanish, and Portuguese, foster communication, training, and debate among individuals and institutions. The range of issues tackled: reforming processes, managing essential public health functions, and developing schools of public health.

Source: Boelen 2000; www.the-networktufh.org; www.campusvirtualsp.org/eng/.

programs, short-term training, and distance learning. Continuous learning can also underpin certification and other professional validation mechanisms. Worker efforts to maintain and upgrade competencies should be recognized and rewarded by career opportunities.

The activity of greatest potential in low-income countries is short-term in-service training. To align it with national workforce plans and priorities requires linking training to supervision, support, and priority program development—and avoiding ad hoc, episodic, fragmented activities. Learners should see short-term training as part of their career development. Pedagogic methods can also improve the productivity of training. The "Health Workers for Change" project illustrates the creative use of participatory methods, including role playing, proactive learning, drama and poetry, and other modalities of unconventional learning.[54]

The internet has extended access to information, lowered costs, and enabled even remotely posted workers to stay connected to information and knowledge. The major drawback of earlier distance education was the lack of discussion and exchange among students and teachers. This appears to have been overcome by email and electronic conferencing. The internet also offers potential for strengthening health information systems.

The internet and email are also providing up-to-date information for health professionals. Cuba's health information network, Infomed, links all of Cuba's hospitals and polyclinics, health research institutions, pharmaceutical production facilities, and local doctors' offices, helping users identify and share low-cost solutions to health and medical problems. It has increased interaction among Cuba's medical and health workers, the public, and the global health

> **Leaders can create change in the midst of uncertainty, address ingrained organizational cultures, and manage constraints that are sometimes beyond their direct control**

Box 3.4 | Professional associations as partners

Professional associations are formally organized groups of individuals or organizations with common professional interests, working together for the benefit of society and for their professions.

The stark contrasts in health needs across the world are linking professional associations in new strategic alliances and in partnerships with the public, for-profit, and not-for-profit sectors to improve the health of the world's people. For example, the World Health Professions Alliance—an alliance of the International Council of Nurses, the World Medical Association, and the International Pharmaceutical Federation—is working with governments, policymakers, and the World Health Organization to deliver cost-effective, quality healthcare worldwide. The alliance of nurses, physicians, and pharmacists also works with other associations of midwives, dentists, and physical therapists on such issues as equity and access to health care, human resource planning (to ensure right numbers with right qualifications), and roles and scope of practice.

Professional councils and associations are particularly important in countries because they participate in the certification, accreditation, and regulation of medical practices. They also uphold the ethical and professional standards of practice, even as they naturally protect the self-interests of their membership. International federations of these national bodies can be extremely helpful in intractable national debates by disseminating best practices and progressive contributions of these professional bodies to global health equity. Such international facilitation is especially important in skill delegation, salary negotiations, regulations and legislation, and migration policies.

Source: International Council of Nurses 1996.

---

community. It is also available to Cuban medical teams and experts providing free health assistance in 14 countries in Africa, Asia, and Latin America.

Fostering leadership and entrepreneurship. Wherever successful workforce development occurs, local leadership can be credited. Nurturing leadership skills can enable workers to collaborate in teams, diagnose new situations, listen to others, and take risks. Leaders can create change in the midst of uncertainty, address ingrained organizational cultures, and manage constraints that are sometimes beyond their direct control. Educational programs that successfully nurture these attributes include team-oriented problem-solving exercises, supervised follow-up, structured mentoring and technical assistance, and networking for resource sharing. Leadership takes time—and sustained efforts—to develop. A successful leadership education model, for instance, might include multiple short-term engagements over 12–18 months, with supervised work activities.[55]

Health leadership and management training should be part of strategic human resource development. A global learning forum on health leadership and management could be created to share good practices, improve monitoring and evaluation, and encourage collaborative opportunities. Explicit attempts should be made to close the gender gap in health leadership by recruiting women for such training programs. At the national and subregional levels, health leadership

❝❝ Health workforce development requires as much policy support from outside the health sector as from within

and management centers could be created to strengthen institutional leadership capacity.

Professional and peer systems, the keepers of the health professions, can strengthen technical quality, standards, ethics, leadership behavior, and camaraderie. They are vital for regulation, monitoring, and data gathering, especially for the private sector, where few other controls of practitioners exist. But professional associations are also interest groups and lobbying groups, protecting and raising the compensation and status of their members (box 3.4). International associations of professionals can align professional accreditation systems so that appropriate learning is promoted and rewarded.

Developing enabling policies

Health workforce development requires as much policy support from outside the health sector as from within. Macroeconomic policies set the bounds for what is possible in the overall budget and in the health budget. Decisions in the civil service and the ministries of finance, education, labor, and planning also shape the workforce environment. Without their cooperation, the health sector is comparatively powerless to plan and manage its workforce. (Migration policies, also important, are addressed in the next chapter.)

Macroeconomic policies

Workforce development depends on public spending to create posts, pay salaries, and finance incentives. Supportive macroeconomic policies are thus essential for workforce development. Yet many countries are only now emerging from demoralizing hiring caps and salary freezes. Bans on recruitment and staffing are still in force in many countries, and

in others the public expenditure budgets are still highly restrictive. Even with severe worker shortages, countries with a wage bill that is considered beyond affordability face continuing staff cuts.

In some countries, there is an urgent priority to rapidly scale up life-saving interventions. Donors are proposing large infusions of funds. Grant funds to address HIV/AIDS, estimated at $5 billion in 2003, are projected to continue to increase over the next five years.[56] Yet many ministries of finance have imposed macroeconomic public expenditure ceilings with employment and wage caps. Without lifting these ceilings, workforce expansion, salary improvements, and incentive payments will be impossible.

Some claim that these ceilings are part of the "conditionality" imposed by international financial institutions. Finance officials worry about the negative effects of the massive inflow of donor funds, causing fiscal volatility, unsustainable debt, currency appreciation and inflation—a variant of the "Dutch disease" that can plague oil exporters when they receive sudden windfalls. They also worry about expanding off-budget expenditures. Others argue that countries' lack of absorptive capacity and the lack of sustained donor involvement and harmonization compromise the usefulness of large infusions of funds.

How can "workforce-friendly" macroeconomic policies be created? To begin, perceptions and attitudes must change. Whether budgetary ceilings are real or not, many believe that caps exist, and many officials have been accustomed to ceilings, especially on social expenditures. The situation parallels a family with a severely sick member. Costly life-saving medical care is necessary but not affordable. The family is prepared to spend heavily,

" Many countries face very tough choices. Spending at unsustainable levels can be wasteful and unproductive, yet without financing for workforce development, many lives will be lost

even incurring large debts, to save a life. What does a country do under similar circumstances?

Many countries face very tough choices. Spending at unsustainable levels can be wasteful and unproductive. Yet without financing for workforce development, many lives will be lost. The decisions clearly belong to the societies and citizens who have to incur the risks and command the benefits. A participatory process that engages key stakeholders is essential to harmonize national health priorities and macroeconomic policies. Much like the policy appeals for "structural adjustment with a human face" in the 1980s, we must craft new "macroeconomic policies for saving lives" in our time.

Several international initiatives—including the Heavily Indebted Poor Countries (HIPC) Initiative, the poverty reduction strategy papers (PRSPs), and sector-wide approaches (SWAps)—offer an opportunity for countries to use the macroeconomic policy environment to promote the health workforce. The key is not necessarily to spend more on the workforce, but to spend more effectively. And more effective spending on the health workforce hinges on the sector-wide coordination of resources allocated to human resources for health.

Important for this coordination are a health workforce strategic plan that lays out national health workforce policy priorities and a health workforce expenditure plan that coordinates and guides resource allocation.[57] These plans can set priorities for health workforce issues within health and across other key sectors, through PRSPs, SWAps, and other tools available to developing countries. PRSPs lay emphasis on the health sector and highlight key actions. SWAps bring together governments, development partners, and other stakeholders to

develop health sector strategies and programs. Using these macroeconomic mechanisms to make national expenditures on the health workforce more coherent and strategic in the long term promises high returns to national investments in health workers.

Educational policies

Sound national primary and secondary educational systems are often overlooked in the production of health workers. These are the foundations for the training of allied professionals and technical workers. Another foundation is higher education, with its medical, nursing, dental, and pharmacy schools. In some countries, situating responsibility for medical education in the ministry of health has been an effective way to improve the linkages between the various levels of education and the health education system. This has also improved the fit between health education and health system needs in countries, as in Iran (box 3.5).

Educational policies can also ensure that education is aligned with the health needs of the population. The ministries of education, health, finance, and others—including women, minority groups, indigenous peoples—can enhance the diversity of the health student body and build a health system that increases social and geographic access. Improving the recruitment of students from underserved populations, broadening the financing of educational opportunities to rural and remote areas, and providing financing options for students from low-income backgrounds can all help in this.

Educational policies can, in addition, promote regular review or reform of health professions curricula, improving the orientation to community and population needs while deemphasizing

Box
3.5 | **Iran's revolution in health**

In 1985 Iran established a national Ministry of Health and Medical Education to improve the country's development of human resources for health and to better match health education to population health needs. There has been enormous progress in ensuring the availability of a health workforce with the right number and skill mix of workers.

The ministry is responsible for all aspects of planning, leadership, supervision, and evaluation of health services, including the training and educating of human resources for health, within the "Comprehensive Health Delivery System" that makes up Iran's health infrastructure. Human resource development, training, and education are overseen by three undersecretaries in the ministry.

The Undersecretary for Health Affairs directly oversees the training of community health workers, or behvarzes, and female volunteers. Behvarzes, both male and female, are selected from local rural populations, trained in Behvarz Educational Centers, and staff rural health houses. The number of behvarzes is determined by the size of the rural population, and 32,500 trained behvarzes are currently delivering services in health houses.

The Undersecretary for Educational and Universities Affairs is responsible for educating and training

health professionals and ensuring continuing education programs. From 1985 to 2000 the number of medical students increased by approximately 27,000, and the number of other health profession students by approximately 60,000.

The Office of Continuing Education—working with 44 universities and faculties, 62 scientific-professional associations, and 10 research centers—directs continuing education programs for all licensed medical staff in Iran, including physicians, dentists, pharmacists, and lab technicians. In 1998, 908 such programs were administered; in 2001, 1,505.

The Ministry also has an Undersecretary for Management and Resources Development and Parliamentary Affairs, directly responsible for training managers and employees. Training programs

are tailored to target groups with the goal of maintaining standards and continuously improving academic knowledge among managers and employees. At the end of all courses, attendees receive a license and after completing 176 hours of training they receive an additional monetary bonus.

Iran's innovative integration of medical education and the health care system has dramatically expanded access to health services throughout the country, reduced reliance on external workers and services, and significantly improved key health indicators (see table).

Iran's Ministry of Health and Medical Education has attracted considerable attention around the world and has been cited by the former chief of the World Federation of Medical Education as a model appropriate for the 21st century.

Large gains from integrating medical education and the health care system in Iran

Indicator	1984	2000
Physicians	14,000	70,000
Physicians per 1,000 population	0.39	1.04
Full-time faculty members	3,153	9,000
Ratio of students in postdoctoral programs to all medical students (%)	2.3	10.0
Infant mortality rate (per 1,000 live births)	51	26
Under-five mortality rate	70	33
Vaccination coverage against 7 contagious diseases (%)	20	95
Patients sent abroad for treatment	11,000	200
Foreign medical workers	3,153	0

Source: Vatankhah 2002.

competitiveness on the international labor market. With regular curriculum reviews, a more dynamic learning system can be created to benefit both students and their eventual patients. Many education policies—including recruitment plans and curriculum reform in medical and nursing education—require long-term investments, with payoffs coming after lags of several years.

Workforce development in health should thus be part of national educational policies. Policies to protect, support, and value both medical workers and teachers can be applied in both sectors. Joint advocacy could also help both sectors—their public allocations tend to rise and fall together—garner public support for more social expenditure by the government.

Civil service reform

Public health workers are usually part of a nation's civil service, which many countries have been reforming, usually through downsizing, severance, new wage scales, and realigned benefits. Successful reforms require ownership by all stakeholders and sensitivity to those who lose out. They require vision, stamina, and institutional capacity.

A major question is whether health workers should be delinked from other civil servants, as Uganda and Ghana are considering. Some argue that health workers should remain part of the civil service. Their separation would cause resentment among others, and pressures for special treatment would soon build from teachers, administrators, and other civil servants. Others argue that health workers could be brought together as a medical cadre in public service. They see health work as different and distinctive, because they are attracted to highly competitive

labor markets in the private sector and overseas and because they perform life-saving functions.

Private sector

The public sector in health can learn from many of the innovative approaches and successful efforts in the private sector. A new health franchise initiative has been proposed in Kenya to deliver tuberculosis and HIV/AIDS services through decentralized, self-financed units expanded through the private sector. New mixes of public-private partnerships also show promise. Tanzania's Kilimanjaro Christian Medical Center is privately operated but publicly funded under state contract. And in Mali decentralization is leading to public-private partnerships, with local communities contracting, hiring, firing, and paying health workers. Governments are also contracting work out to the private sector.[58]

The quality in the private sector is often uncertain, particularly for diseases requiring long-term treatment.[59] Private sector care for tuberculosis is associated with a 9–10 week delay in starting appropriate treatment, worrisome because the costs of delay are society-wide.[60] The unregulated and variable use of antiretroviral therapy for HIV/AIDS and mono-therapy treatments for tuberculosis among private providers in Africa have led to fears of rapid increases in multidrug resistance strains of both diseases.[61]

Although many global health goals will be hard to reach without engaging the private sector, incentives and systems need to be in place to assure the delivery of standard quality health care. If the private sector provides quality services at reasonable prices, there is every reason to promote and encourage its growth and development. Government has the instruments to

Box 3.6	**Human resources in transitional economies**

A WHO/Euro survey in 2000 concluded that eastern European countries confront shared human resources problems of shortages, over-supply, distributional imbalances, migration, inadequate incentives to motivate workers, and weak planning and management. Worker shortages are pronounced for elderly care, while oversupply, especially of physicians, is common. All countries experience urban concentration and suffer from weak rural coverage. With the growth of private for-profit health care, the most talented and competitive workers are shifting from public to private sectors. With the expansion of the European Union, workers are also migrating from poorer eastern to richer western European countries.

Much of the imbalance is due to economic and political transitions from socialism to capitalism, impacting both the supply and demand for health services. Most countries are only beginning to develop national plans to cope with workforce challenges. Among key human resource strategies are managing the public-private mix, improving the work environment, enhancing educational relevance and quality, revamping professional accreditation and regulation, and developing recruitment, retention, and return strategies.

Source: Kaunas University of Medicine 2004.

do this—with information, regulation, licensing, taxation, and incentives. Another important instrument is peer oversight by professional associations.

Learning for improvement

Strategic planning and management of the workforce is an iterative process of action, learning, and adjustment. Setbacks and progress are inherent in the process, and adjustments need to be continually implemented for steady improvement.

What is needed for countries to adopt the five-dimensional approach proposed here? Political commitment is a key element in all successful workforce reforms.[62] When decisionmakers are frequently replaced and priorities redefined, it may be difficult to devise policies with a long-term perspective. Examples of strong political commitment leading to effective human resources for health policies, are Brazil (family health program), Iran (rural health program),

and Thailand, which has engaged consistently in human resources policy for 40 years.[63]

Also critical is learning what works and what doesn't. Progress and setbacks must be tracked. Lessons about better (and worse) practices must be learned. Monitoring and evaluation must trigger a virtuous cycle of learning improvements and complete the loop of planning, implementation, and continuous improvement.

Monitoring and evaluation require metrics of workforce performance to assess and track developments and to guide downstream adjustments. The recent fad for results-based monitoring, while useful, should be broadened to strengthen practical action. Tracking results keeps the focus on goals and intermediate targets. But measuring and monitoring must also track political, economic, social, and managerial processes to determine the reasons for success or failure—and more important—to identify what can be done to correct for deficiencies.

> **“** Countries, alone or in collaboration, must strengthen their capacity for strategic planning, management, and policy development

This learning and feedback demand a critical mass of leaders and technicians with relevant technical competencies. Countries, alone or in collaboration, must strengthen their capacity for strategic planning, management, and policy development. The skills required: situational assessment, data collection, analysis of the policy context, identifying options and determining their feasibility, planning and policy development, and mobilizing and leading stakeholders through the workforce development process.

Capacity building for health system planners and managers, although very important and desirable, can also be difficult to develop. In some countries there is a coexistence of shortages in planning and management positions with unfilled vacancies. Many countries lack the capacity to absorb donor funding, reflecting past underinvestments. But they also lack financing to build national capacity. The symptom? Committed yet unspent grant funds. The cause? Weak public expenditure management systems—lacking the budget, administration, and skills to effectively manage grants.

Conclusion

A five-dimensional strategic approach—engaging stakeholders, planning human investments, managing for performance, developing enabling policies, and learning for improvement—can help to energize national action on the health workforce.

Because health challenges and resources vary across contexts, each country should take the five strategic dimensions detailed throughout this chapter and develop an action plan crafted to its own workforce patterns and pace of change. Within any cluster of countries is considerable scope for positive or negative deviance, so that

even countries with low worker density can achieve enormous efficiency gains by adopting an appropriate strategic response and supporting it with effective leadership and political commitment.

The strategic management of human resources is crucial. For example, Malawi is able to achieve, with one-fifth the worker density of Nigeria, the same under-five mortality as Nigeria. Although Kenya spends about the same amount on health as Côte d'Ivoire, it has almost double the health worker density and a far better under-five mortality rate. Honduras and El Salvador have the same under-five mortality level although worker density in Honduras is only half that of El Salvador. These contrasts hold out the promise that better workforce planning and management can generate high health returns, even within limited budgets. In other words, countries can attain significant efficiency gains by improving workforce performance even without shifting to a significantly different worker density.

Many of the challenges facing national actors in workforce development—whether in terms of retaining health workers, accessing necessary inputs, or investing in appropriate education and training—are affected by processes beyond the local and national level. Global forces and global actors—among them, transnational NGOs, development partners and international agencies, and multilateral institutions—all play a role. Yet by working together, national and international actors can harness the power of global flows of resources—particularly knowledge, people, and financing—to strengthen national health workforces and promote global health equity.

Notes
1. Wibulpolprasert and Pengpaibon 2003.

2. Campos 2004.
3. Vatankhah 2002.
4. Martinez and Collini 1999.
5. Luz 1994.
6. Hall 1998.
7. O'Brien-Pallas and others 2001; Bloor and others 2003.
8. Hargadon and Plsek 2004.
9. World Bank 2004a.
10. Tudor Hart 1971.
11. Many frameworks have been proposed for human resources for health. None is automatically superior to another, and this framework contains strategic elements of several other frameworks. Its structure, however, has been simplified to present numerous workforce strategies together in a coherent manner.
12. For Brazil, Colombia, and Thailand, data compiled by the Joint Learning Initiative from WHO 2004. For Central and Eastern European countries and Commonwealth of Independent States countries, see Saltman and Figueras (1997, p. 240).
13. Preker and Feachem 1994.
14. Zaidi 1986; Doescher and others 2000; Chaudhury and Hammer 2003.
15. Canadian Institute for Health Information 2003.
16. Other methodologies result in similarly large estimates of quantitative gaps for severe deficit countries. See Kurowski and others (2003).
17. Narasimhan 2002.
18. OECD 2004.
19. Buchan and Dal Poz 2002.
20. Svitone and others 2000.
21. Vaz and others 1999.
22. Dovlo 2004.
23. Egger and others 2000.
24. Dovlo 2004.
25. Taylor 1992.
26. Lyons 2004.
27. Rigoli and Dussault 2003.
28. Chomitz and others 1998; Wibulpolprasert 1999; Wibulpolprasert and Pengpaibon 2003.
29. Chomitz and others 1998; Hammer and Jack 2002.
30. Quoted in Walker and Gilson (2004, p. 1257).
31. Ferrinho and others 2004; Vujicic and others 2004.
32. Codija and Ouoba 2003.
33. Fikru 2004.
34. ILO and WHO 2002.
35. Ferrinho and others 2003; Ijumba 2003.
36. Ijumba 2003.
37. Habte 2002.
38. Wibulpolprasert and Pengpaibon 2003.
39. Chowdhury 2003.
40. Ferrinho and others 2004.
41. Mathauer and Imhoff 2004.
42. Wagstaff and Claeson 2004.
43. Standing and Baume 2001.
44. Reinikka and Svensson 2003.
45. Kaseje 2004.
46. Mathauer and Imhoff 2004.
47. ILO and WHO 2002.
48. ICN 2003.
49. WHO 2000.
50. Ijsselmuiden 2003.
51. Ndumbe 2004.
52. Boufford 2004.
53. Neufeld and Johnson 2004.
54. Vlassoff and Fonn 2001.
55. Boufford 2004.
56. UNAIDS 2004.
57. Kurowski 2004.
58. Marek 1999; Loevinsohn 2002.
59. Somse and others 2000; Schneider and others 2001; Chabikuli and others 2002.
60. Needham and others 2001.
61. Brugha 2003.
62. Saltman and Figueras 1997.
63. Wibulpolprasert and Pengpaibon 2003.

References

Adams, Orvill. 2002. "WHO Perspective on Human Resources for Health: Consultation on Imbalances in the Health Workforce: Conceptual and Practical Challenges." World Health Organization, Geneva.

Africa News. 2003a. "Nurses Strike to Demand Protection from Contagious Disease." November 25.

———. 2003b. "Nurses Strike Legal— Trade Union." September 23.

———. 2004a. "Hospital Strike Forces Hundreds of Patients to Go Home." January 30.

———. 2004b. "Resident Doctors Begin Strike." February 25.

Aitken, Jean-Marion, and Julia Kemp. 2003. "HIV/AIDS, Equity, and Health Sector Personnel in Southern Africa." Discussion Paper 12. EQUINET, Harare.

Alwan, A., and P. Hornby. 2002. "The Implications of Health Sector Reform for Human Resources Development." *Bulletin of the World Health Organization* 80 (1): 56–60.

Armstrong, Sue. 2000. *Caring for Carers: Managing Stress in Those Who Care for People with HIV and AIDS.* Geneva: Joint United Nations Programme on HIV/AIDS.

Awases M., A. Gbary, J. Nyoni, and R. Chatora. 2003. "Migration of Health Professionals in Six Countries: A Synthesis Report." World Health Organization, Regional Office for Africa, District Health Systems, Brazzaville.

Bandaranayake, D. 2001. "Assessing Performance Management of Human Resources for Health in South-East Asian Countries: Aspects of Quality and Outcome." Paper presented at the World Health Organization Workshop on Global Health Workforce Strategy, Annecy, France, December 9–12, 2000.

Bansal, R. K. 2003. "Private Medical Education Takes Off in India." *The Lancet* 361 (9370): 1748–49.

Bennett, Sarah, and Lynne Miller Franco. 1999. "Public Sector Health Worker Motivation and Health Sector Reform: A Conceptual Framework." Major Applied Research 5, Technical Paper 1. Partnerships for Health Reform Project, Bethesda, Md.

Bennett, Sarah, David Gzirishvili, and Ruth Kanfer. 2000. "An In-depth Analysis of the Determinants and Consequences of Worker Motivation in Two Hospitals in Tbilisi, Georgia." Major Applied Research 5, Working Paper 9. Partnerships for Health Reform, Bethesda, Md.

Bennett, Sarah, Lynne Miller Franco, Ruth Kanfer, and Patrick Stubblebine. 2001. "The Development of Tools to Measure the Determinants and Consequences of Health Worker Motivation in Developing Countries." Major Applied Research 5, Technical Paper 2. Partnerships for Health Reform, Bethesda, Md.

Bennett, S., and E. Ngalande-Banda. 1994. "Public and Private Roles in Health: A Review and Analysis of Experience in Sub-Saharan Africa." ARA Paper Number 6. World Health Organization, Geneva.

Bertrand, William E., Seth Berkeley, and Susan Janoski. 1997. "The Public Health School Without Walls Project: New Models of Public Health Education." *New York Health Sciences Journal* 2 (1): 17–34.

Berwick, D. M. 2002. "A Learning World for the Global Fund." *British Medical Journal* 325 (7355): 55–56.

Bhat, R. 1996. "Regulating the Private Health Care Sector: The Case of the Indian Consumer Protection Act." *Health Policy Plan* 11 (3): 265–79.

Biscoe, Gillian. 2001. "Human Resources: The Political and Policy Context." Prepared for the Global Health Workforce Strategy Group. World Health Organization, Geneva.

Bloor, K., A. Maynard, J. Hall, P. Ulmann, O. Farhauer, and B. Lindgren. 2003. "Planning Human Resources in Health Care—Towards an Economic Approach: An International Comparative Review." Canadian Health Services Research Foundation, Toronto, Canada.

Boelen, Charles. 2000. "Towards Unity for Health: Challenges and Opportunities for Partnership in Health Development." Working Paper. World Health Organization, Geneva.

———. 2002. "A New Paradigm for Medical Schools a Century after Flexner's Report." *Bulletin of the World Health Organization* 80 (7): 592–602.

Boonyoen, Damrong. 1997. "Health Systems and Human Resources Development: The Changing Roles of Public and Private Sectors." *Human Resources for Health Development Journal* 1 (1): 13–18.

Boufford, J. I. 2004. "Leadership Development for Global Health." Joint Learning Initiative Working Paper. New York University, New York. [www.globalhealthtrust.org/].

Brugha, R. 2003. "Antiretroviral Treatment in Developing Countries: The Peril of Neglecting Private Providers." *British Medical Journal* 326 (7403): 1382–84.

Brugha, R., and A. Zwi. 1998. "Improving the Quality of Private Sector Delivery of Public Health Services: Challenges and Strategies." *Health Policy and Planning* 13 (2): 107–20.

Buchan, James, and Mario R. Dal Poz. 2002. "Skill Mix in the Healthcare Workforce: Reviewing the Evidence." *Bulletin of the World Health Organization* 80 (7): 575–80.

Buckley, R., and J. Caple. 2004. *The Theory and Practice of Training.* London: Kogan Page.

Campos, Francisco, José Roberto Ferreira, Maria Fátima de Souza, and Raphael Augusto Teixeira de Aguiar. 2004. "The Innovations on Human Resources Development and the Role of Community Health Workers." Universidade Federal de Minas Gerais Núcleo de Pesquisa em Saúde Coletiva, Brazil. Joint Learning Initiative Working Paper. [www.globalhealthtrust.org/].

Canadian Institute for Health Information. 2003. *Health Indicators.* Ontario.

Chabikuli N., H. Schneider, D. Blaauw, A. B. Zwi, and R. Brugha. 2002. "Quality and Equity of Private Sector Care for Sexually Transmitted Diseases in South Africa." *Health Policy and Planning* 17 (Suppl.): 40–46.

Chaudhury, Nzamul, and Jeffrey S. Hammer. 2003. "Ghost Doctors: Absenteeism in Bangladeshi Health Facilities." Policy Research Working Paper 3065. World Bank, Development Research Group, Washington, D.C. [Retrieved October 6, 2004, from http://econ.worldbank.org/files/27031_wps3065.pdf].

Chomitz, Kenneth M., Gunawan Setiadi, Azrul Azwar, Nusye Ismail, and Widiyarti. 1998. "What Do Doctors Want? Developing Incentives for Doctors to Serve in Indonesia's Rural and Remote Areas." Policy Research Working Paper 1888. World Bank,

Washington, D.C. [Retrieved October 6, 2004, from http://econ.worldbank.org/docs/303.pdf].

Chowdhury, Mustaque. 2003. "Health Workforce for TB Control by DOTS: The BRAC Case." Joint Learning Initiative Working Paper. BRAC, Bangladesh. [www.globalhealthtrust.org/].

Chunaras, S. 1998. "Human Resources for Health Planning: A Review of the Thai Experience." *Human Resources Development Journal* 2(2).

Classoff, C., and S. Fonn. 2001. "Health Workers for Change as a Health Systems Management and Development Tool." *Health Policy and Planning* 16 (Suppl. 1): 47–52.

Codjia Laurence, and V. Ouoba. 2003. "Motivation des personnels de sante, Rapport Final." Burkina Faso Ministry of Health and World Health Organization. Burkina Faso.

Demery, Lionel, Shiyan Chao, Ren Bernier, and Kalpana Mehra. 1995. "The Incidence of Social Spending in Ghana." PSP Discussion Paper 82. World Bank, Poverty and Social Policy Department, Washington, D.C.

Deutsche Presse-Agentur. 2003a. "Politician Turns Mortician to Cope with Hospital Strike in Sri Lanka." September 22.

———. 2003b. "Ecuador's Embattled Gutierrez Freezes Public Wages amid Unrest." December 18.

Dewdney, John. 2001. *WHO/RTC Health Workforce Planning Workbook*. Center for Public Health, University of New South Wales, Sydney. [Retrieved October 14, 2004, from http://hrhtoolkit.forumone. com/planania/mstr_planania_workbook.pdf].

Di Martino, V. 2002. *Workplace Violence in the Health Sector—Country Case Studies Brazil, Bulgaria, Lebanon, Portugal, South Africa, Thailand, plus an Additional Australian Study: Synthesis Report*. Geneva: ILO/ICN/WHO/PSI Joint Programme on Workplace Violence in the Health Sector.

Doescher, M. P., K. E. Ellsbury, and L. G. Hart. 2000. "The Distribution of Rural Female Generalist Physicians in the United States." *Journal of Rural Health* 16 (2): 111–18.

Dovlo, Delanyo. 1998. "Health Sector Reform and Deployment, Training and Motivation of Human Resources towards Equity in Health Care: Issues and Concerns in Ghana." *Human Resources Development Journal* 2(1). [Retrieved October 6, 2004, from www. moph.go.th/ops/hrdj/Hrdj_no3/manila6.doc].

———. 2004. "Using Mid-Level Cadres as Substitutes for Internationally Mobile Health Professionals in Africa. A Desk Review." *Human Resources for Health* 2(7).

Dussault, Gilles. 1999. "Human Resources Development: The Challenge for Health Sector Reform." The Fourth Adapting to Change Global Core Course on Population, Reproductive Health and Health Sector Reform, August 19–30, 2002, ILO Training Center, Turin, Italy. World Bank. [Retrieved October 6, 2004, from www.reprohealth.org/ turin_part/Week2/2Tue27/Ses5/Reading2.pdf].

Dussault, Gilles, and Carl-Ardy Dubois. 2003. "Human Resources for Health Policies: A Critical Component in Health Policies." *Human Resources for Health* 1(1).

Dussault, Gilles, and Maria Christina Franceschini. 2003. "Not Enough Here, Too Many There: Understanding Geographical Imbalances in the Distribution of Health Personnel." World Bank, Washington, D.C.

Eckhert, N. L. 2002. "The Global Pipeline: Too Narrow, Too Wide or Just Right?" *Medical Education* 36 (7): 606–13.

Egger, Dominique, Debra Lipson, and Orvill Adams. 2000. "Achieving the Right Balance: The Role of Policy-Making Processes in Managing Human Resources for Health Problems." Issues in Health Services Delivery Discussion Paper 2. World Health Organization, Geneva.

Fabricant, S. J., C. W. Kamara, and A. Mills. 1999. "Why the Poor Pay More: Household Curative Expenditures in Rural Sierra Leone." *International Journal of Health Planning and Management* 14 (4): 339–40.

Fee, E., and B. Rosenkrantz. 1991. "Professional Education for Public Health in the United States." In *A History of Education in Public Health*. Oxford: Oxford University Press.

Ferrinho, P., A. Biscaia, I. Vronteira, I. Craveiro, A. Antunes, C. Conceicao, I. Flores, and O. Santos. 2003. "Patterns of Perceptions of Workplace Violence in the Portuguese Health Care Sector." *Human Resources for Health* 1(11). [Retrieved October 6, 2004, from www.human-resources-health.com/content/1/1/11].

Ferrinho, Paulo, Wim Van Lerberghe, Ines Fronteira, and Fatima Hipolito Ba Soc. 2004. "Dual Practice in the Health Sector." Joint Learning Initiative Working Paper. Garcia de Orta Development and Cooperation Association, Portugal; World Health Organization, Geneva. [www.globalhealthtrust.org/].

Fikru, Bruck. 2004. "Toward Developing Policy for Human Resources for Health in Ethiopia (While Facing the Challenge of Meeting the MDGs for Child Survival)." Report for United Nations Children's Fund, Addis Ababa.

Financial Times. 2004. "Health Strike Adds to Berlusconi Problems." February 10.

Franco, Lynne, Sara Bennett, and Ruth Kanfer. 2002. "Health Sector Reform and Public Sector Health Worker Motivation: A Conceptual Framework." *Social Science and Medicine* 54 (8): 1255–66.

Fraser, Sarah W., and Trisha Greenhalgh. 2001.

"Coping with Complexity: Educating for Capability."
British Medical Journal 323 (7316): 799–803.

Goudge, Jane. 1999. "The Public-Private Mix." In Nicholas
Crisp, ed., *South African Health Review 1999*. Durban:
Health Systems Trust. [www.hst.org.za/sahr].

Grant, K., and R. Grant. 2003. "Health Insurance
and the Poor in Low Income Countries." *World
Hospital and Health Services* 39 (1): 19–22.

Gruen, Reinhold, Raqibul Anwar, Tahmina Begum, James R.
Killingsworth, and Charles Normand. 2002. "Dual Job
Holding Practitioners in Bangladesh: An Exploration."
Social Science and Medicine 54 (2): 267–79.

Ha, N. T., P. Berman, and U. Larsen. 2002.
"Household Utilization and Expenditure on
Private and Public Health Services in Vietnam."
Health Policy and Planning 17 (1): 61–70.

Habte, Demissie. 2002. "The Crisis of Human Resources
for Health Research and Health Care: A Call for Action."
Plenary session on Monitoring the Results of Research
Capacity Strengthening, 14 November, Arusha. Global
Forum for Health Research. [Retrieved October 6, 2004,
from www.globalforumhealth.org/forum_6/sessions/
3Thursday/7Plenary6MonitoringHabteFull.doc].

Hall, Thomas L. 1998. "Why Plan Human Resources
for Health?" *Human Resources for Health
Development Journal* 2 (2): 77–86.

Hammer, Jeffrey, and William Jack. 2002. "The Design
of Incentives for Health Care Providers in Developing
Countries: Contracts, Competition and Cost-Control."
Journal of Development Economics 69 (1): 297–303.

Hanson, Kara, and Peter Berman. 1998. "Private
Health Care Provision in Developing Countries: A
Preliminary Analysis of Levels and Composition."
Health Policy and Planning 13 (3): 195–211.

Hargadon, Judy, and Paul Plsek. 2004. "Complexity and
Health Workforce Issues." Joint Learning Initiative
Working Paper. New Ways of Working Modernisation
Agency, United Kingdom; Paul E. Plsek & Associates,
United Kingdom. [www.globalhealthtrust.org/].

Hicks, Vern, and Orvill Adams. 2001. "Pay and Non-
Pay Incentives, Performance and Motivation."
Prepared for the Global Health Workforce Strategy
Group, World Health Organization, Geneva.

ICN (International Council of Nurses). 1996.
"Professional and Socio-Economic Welfare
Responsibilities within NNAs." Geneva.

———. 2003. "Novel AIDS Treatment Programme
for Health Care Workers in Zambia." ICN
Press Release, November 13, Geneva.

Ijsselmuiden, Carel. 2003. "Training of Health Care

Workers. Graduate Education in Public Health:
AfriHealth Survey: Provisional Results and
Conclusions." Draft. Prepared for the Joint Learning
Intiative, September 29–October 3, Accra.

Ijumba, P. 2003. "'Voices' of Primary Health Care
Facility Workers." In P. Ijumba, A. Ntuli, and
P. Barron, eds., *South African Health Review
2002*. Durban: Health Systems Trust.

Illawarra Mercury. 2003. "Hospital Strike
Causes Chaos." October 8.

ILO (International Labour Organization). 1999. Terms of
Employment and Working Conditions in Health Sector
Reforms: Report for discussion at the Joint Meeting on
Terms of Employment and Working Conditions in Health
Sector Reforms. Geneva: International Labour Office.
[Retrieved October 6, 2004, from www.ilo.org/public/
english/dialogue/sector/techmeet/jmhsr98/jmhsrr.htm].

ILO (International Labour Organization) and WHO
(World Health Organizaiton). 2002. "Framework
Guidelines for Addressing Workplace
Violence in the Health Sector." Geneva.

International Nursing Foundation of Japan. 2000.
Nursing in the World. Tokyo: Kudan-Kita.

Kanyesigye, Edward, and G. M. Ssendyona. 2003. "Payment
of Lunch Allowance: A Case Study of the Uganda
Health Service." Joint Learning Initiative Working
Paper. Ministry of Health, Uganda. Ministry of Public
Service, Uganda. [www.globalhealthtrust.org/].

Kaseje, Dan. 2004. "Community Involvement in Health
Professionals' Education to Strengthen Them for
their Role in Strengthening Health Care Systems
in Africa." Joint Learning Initiative Working Paper.
The Tropical Institute of Community Health and
Development, Kenya. [www.globalhealthtrust.org/].

Kaunas University of Medicine. 2004. "Developing
an Effective Health Sector Workforce."
Proceedings of a regional expert consultation
workshop, February 13, Lithuania.

Kolehmainen-Aitken, Riitta-Liisa. 2004. "Decentralization's
Impact on the Health Workforce: Perspectives
of Managers, Workers and National Leaders."
Human Resources for Health 2(5).

Kortenbout, Elma. 1998. "Production of Nurses in
South Africa." In Antoinette Ntuli, ed., *South
African Health Review 1998*. Durban: Health
Systems Trust. [www.hst.org.za/sahr].

Kurowski, Christoph. 2004. "Scope, Characteristics and
Policy Implications of the Health Worker Shortage
in Low Income Countries of Sub-Saharan Africa."
Joint Learning Initiative Working Paper. World Bank,

Washington, D.C. [www.globalhealthtrust.org/].

Kurowski, Christoph, and Anne Mills. 2003. "NCTP: A New Method to Estimate Human Resource Requirements in the Context of Scaling Up Priority Interventions." Working Paper. London School of Hygiene and Tropical Medicine.

Kurowski, Christoph, Kaspar Wyss, Salim Abdulla, N'Diekhor Yémadji, and Anne Mills. 2003. "Human Resources for Health: Requirements and Availability in the Context of Scaling-Up Priority Interventions in Low-Income Countries: Case Studies from Tanzania and Chad." Working paper. London School of Hygiene and Tropical Medicine.

Lehmann, Uta, and David Sanders. 1999. "The Production of Doctors." In Nicholas Crisp, ed., *South African Health Review 1999*. Durban: Health Systems Trust. [www.hst.org.za/sahr].

Lerberghe, Wim van, Orvill Adams, and Paulo Ferrinho. 2002. "Human Resources Impact Assessment." *Bulletin of the World Health Organization* 80 (7): 525.

Lethbridge, J. 2002. *Social Dialogue in Health Services: Case Studies in Brazil, Canada, Chile, United Kingdom*. Sectoral Activities Working Paper 189. International Labour Organization, Geneva.

Loevinsohn, B. 2002. *Practical Issues in Contracting for Primary Health Care Delivery: Lessons from Two Large Projects in Bangladesh*. World Bank, Washington, D.C. [Retrieved October 6, 2004, from www. worldbank.org/wbi/healthflagship/oj_ben2.doc].

Lonnroth K., T. U. Tran, L. M. Thuong, H. T. Quy, and V. Diwan. 2001. "Can I Afford Free Treatment? Perceived Consequences of Health Care Provider Choices among People with Tuberculosis in Ho Chi Minh City, Vietnam." *Social Science and Medicine* 52 (6): 935–48.

Luz, M. T. 1994. "As Conferências Nacionais de Saúde e as políticas de saúde da década de 80." In R. Guimarães and R. M. Tavares, eds., *Saúde e Sociedade no Brasil*. Rio de Janeiro: Relume Dumará.

Lyons, Maryinez. 2004. "Health Workers in Uganda: From Crisis to Crisis." Joint Learning Initiative Working Paper. International Organization for Migration, Kenya. [www.globalhealthtrust.org/].

Makan, Bupendra. 1998. "Distribution of Health Personnel." In Antoinette Ntuli, ed., *South African Health Review 1998*. Durban: Health Systems Trust. [www.hst.org.za/sahr].

Marek, T. 1999. "Successful Contracting of Prevention Service: Fighting Malnutrition in Senegal and Madagascar." *Health Policy and Planning* 14(4):382–89.

Martineau, Tim, and James Buchan. 2000. "HR and the Success of Health Sector Reform." 128th Annual Meeting of the American Public Health Association, Eliminating Health Disparities, November 12–16, Boston.

Martineau, Tim, and Javier Martinez. 1997. "Human Resources in the Health Sector: Guidelines for Appraisal and Strategic Development." Health and Development Series, Working Paper 1. European Commission Directorate General for Development, Brussels.

Martinez, J., and L. Collini. 1999. "A Review of Human Resource Issues in the Health Sector: Improving Human Resources as a Step towards Improving the Health Sector." Department for International Development Health Systems Resource Centre, London.

Martinez, Javier, and Tim Martineau. 1998. "Rethinking Human Resources: An Agenda for the Millennium." *Health Policy and Planning* 13 (4): 345–58.

Marzolf, J. 2002. "The Indonesian Private Health Sector: Opportunities for Reform: An Analysis of Obstacles and Constraints to Growth." World Bank, Washington, D.C.

Mathauer, Inke, and Ingo Imhoff. 2004. "Staff Motivation in Central America and Africa: The Impact of Non-Financial Incentives and Quality Management Tools." Draft. Gesellschaft für Technische Zusammenarbeit, Eschborn.

Mercer, Hugo, Mario Dal Poz, Orvill Adams, Barbara Stilwell, James Buchan, Norbert Dreesch, Pascal Zurn, and Robert Beaglehole. 2002. "Human Resources for Health: Developing Policy Options for Change." WHO/EIP/OSD, Geneva. [Retrieved October 6, 2004, from www.who.int/hrh/documents/en/Developing_policy_options.pdf].

Montagu, D., and G. Elzinga. 2004. "Innovations in Access to TB and HIV/AIDS Care in Sub- Saharan Africa: Dynamic Engagement of the Private Sector." *Health Economics and Health Policy*, in press.

Moomal, Hashim, and William Pick. 1998. "Production of Doctors in South Africa." In Antoinette Ntuli, ed., *South African Health Review 1998*. Durban: Health Systems Trust. [www.hst.org.za/sahr].

Moore, M., and A. Tait, eds. 2002. *Open and Distance Learning: Trends, Policy and Strategy Considerations*. United Nations Educational, Scientific and Cultural Organization, Paris.

Mudur, G. 2003. "India Plans to Expand Private Sector in Healthcare Review." *British Medical Journal* 326 (7388): 520.

Mudyarabikwa, Oliver, and Denford Madhina. 2000. "An Assessment of Incentive Setting for Participation of Private For-Profit Health Care Providers in Zimbabwe." Small Applied Research 15. Partnerships for Health Reform, Bethesda, Md.

Mutizwa-Mangiza, D. 1998. "The Impact of Health Sector Reform on Public Sector Health Worker Motivation in

Zimbabwe." Major Applied Research 5, Working Paper 4. Partnerships for Health Reform, Bethesda, Md.

Narasimhan, Vasant. 2002. "Country Case Study: Human Resources for Botswana's National AIDS Treatment Program." Presented at workshop on human resources and national health systems: Shaping the Agenda for Action. World Health Organization, December 2–4, Geneva.

Ndumbe, Peter. 2004. "The Training of Human Resources for Health in Africa." Joint Learning Initiative Working Paper. University of Yaounde, Cameroon. [www. globalhealthtrust.org/]

Needham, D. M., S. D. Foster, G. Tomlinson, and P. Godfrey-Faussett. 2001. "Socio-Economic, Gender and Health Services Factors Affecting Diagnostic Delay for Tuberculosis Patients in Urban Zambia." *Tropical Medicine and International Health* 6 (4): 256–59.

Neufeld, V., and N. Johnson. 2004. "Training and Developing of Health Leaders." Joint Learning Initiative Working Paper. McMaster University, Canada. [www. globalhealthtrust.org/]

Nordin, H. 1995. *Fakta om vaold och hot I arbetet.* Occupational Injury Information System. Swedish Board of Occupational Safety and Health, Solna.

O'Brien-Pallas, L., A. Baumann, G. Donner, G. Tomblin, J. Murphy. 2001. Lochhaas Gerlach, and M. Luba. 2001. "Forecasting Models for Human Resources in Health Care." *Journal of Advanced Nursing* 33 (1): 120–29.

OECD (Organisation for Economic Co-operation and Development). 2004. *Trends in International Migration 2003*. Paris: OECD.

OECD (Organisation for Economic Co-operation and Development), Ad Hoc Group on the OECD Health Project. 2002. "OECD Cross-National Study on 'Human Resources for Health Care (HRHC).'" Progress Report and Issues for Discussion. Experts Meeting, April 10–11, Paris.

Padarath, Ashnie, Charlotte Chamberlain, David McCoy, Antoinette Ntuli, Mike Rowson, and Rene Loewenson. 2003. "Health Personnel in Southern Africa: Confronting Maldistribution and Brain Drain." EQUINET Discussion Paper 4. Harare. [Retrieved October 6, 2004, from ftp:// ftp.hst.org.za/pubs/equity/hrh_review.pdf].

Pan American Health Organization. 1997. "Datos actualizados de Recursos Humanos en Salud en la Region de las Americas." October 7.

Panafrican News Agency. 2003a. "Malian Workers Begin 2-Day Strike." October 6.

———. 2003b. "Workers Down Tools at Zambia's Biggest State Hospital." November 12.

———. 2004. "Aggrieved Zimbabwean Nurses Threaten New Strike." January 22.

Partnerships for Health Reform. Undated. "Using Incentives to Improve Health Care Delivery." PHRplus Issues and Results, Partnerships for Health Reform*plus*, Bethesda, Md.

———. 2001. "Working with Private Providers to Improve the Delivery of Priority Services." PHR Primer for Policymakers, Partnerships for Health Reform, Bethesda, Md.

Preker, A. S., and R. G. A. Feachem. 1994. "Health Care." In N. Barr, ed. 1994. *Labor Markets and Social Policy in Central and Eastern Europe*. Oxford: Oxford University Press.

Pretorius, Engela. 1999. "Traditional Healers." In Nicholas Crisp, ed., *South African Health Review 1999*. Durban: Health Systems Trust. [www.hst.org.za/sahr].

Reid, Steven, and Daphney Conco. 1999. "Monitoring the Implementation of Community Service." In Nicholas Crisp, ed., *South African Health Review 1999*. Durban: Health Systems Trust. [www.hst.org.za/sahr]

Reinikka, Ritva, and Jakob Svensson. 2003. "Working for God? Evaluating Service Delivery of Religious Not-for-Profit Health Care Providers in Uganda." Policy Research Working Paper 3058. World Bank, Washington, D.C.

Rigoli, Felix, and Gilles Dussault. 2003. "The Interface between Health Sector Reform and Human Resources for Health." *Human Resources for Health* 1(9).

Saltman, Richard and Josep Figueras, eds. 1997. *European Health Care Reform: Analysis of Current Strategies*. WHO Regional Office for Europe: Copenhagen.

Scavino, Julio. 2003. "National Disputes in the Health Sector in the Region of the Americas in 2003." Pan American Health Organization, Washington, D.C. [Retrieved October 6, 2004, from www.lachsr.org/observatorio/ eng/policies.html].

Schiavo-Campo, Salvatore, Giulio de Tommaso, and Amitabha Mukherjee. 1997. "Government Employment and Pay in Global Perspective: A Selective Synthesis of International Facts, Policies, and Experience." Policy Research Working Paper 1771. World Bank, Washington, D.C. [Retrieved October 6, 2004, from http://econ. worldbank.org/view.php?type=5&id=895].

Schneider, H., D. Blaauw, E. Dartnall, D. J. Coetzee, and R. C. Ballard. 2001. "STD Care in the South African Private Health Sector." *South African Medical Journal* 91 (2): 151–56.

Somse, P., F. Mberyo-Yaah, P. Morency, M. J. Dubois, G. Gresenguet, and J. Pepin. 2000. "Quality of Sexually Transmitted Disease Treatments in the Formal and

Informal Sectors of Bangui, Central African Republic." *Sexually Transmitted Diseases* 27 (8): 458–64.

South Africa Department of Health. 2001. Department of Health Annual Report April 2000–March 2001. Pretoria. In P. Ijumba, ed., 2003. "'Voices' of Primary Health Care Facility Workers." In P. Ijumba, A. Ntuli, and P. Barron, eds., 2003. *South African Health Review 2002*. Durban: Health Systems Trust.

Standing, Hilary. 2000. "Gender—A Missing Policy Dimension in Human Resource Policy and Planning for Health Reforms." *Human Resources for Health and Development Journal* 4 (1): 2.

Standing, Hilary, and Elaine Baume. 2001. "Equity, Equal Opportunities, Gender and Organization Performance." Workshop on Global Health Workforce Strategy, December 9–12, Annecy, France.

Svitone, E. C., R. Garfield, M. I. Vasconcelos, and V. A. Craveiro. 2000. "Primary Health Care Lessons from the Northeast of Brazil: The Agentes de Saude Program." *Pan American Journal of Public Health* 7 (5): 293–302.

Task Force on Higher Education in Developing Countries. 2000. Higher Education in Developing Countries: Peril and Promise. World Bank, Washington, D.C. [Retrieved October 6, 2004, from www.tfhe.net/report/readreport. htm].

Taylor, J. E. 1992. "Life-Saving Skills Training for Midwives: Report on the Ghanaian Experience." *International Journal of Gynaecology and Obstetrics* 38 (Suppl): S41–43.

Thankappan, K. R., K. Mohandas, Carel Ijsselmuiden, Reginald Matchaba-Hove, and Manju Renjit. 2002. *Public Health Schools without Walls: A Report of Network Activities 2001–2002*. Acutha Menon Centre for Health Science Studies. Thiruvananthapuram, India.

Thaver, Inayat H., Trudy Harpham, Barbara McPake, and Paul Garner. 1998. "Private Practitioners in the Slums of Karachi: What Quality of Care Do They Offer?" *Social Science and Medicine* 46(11):1441–49.

The Times of India. 2004. "Junior Doctors Call Off Strike." January 25.

Tudor Hart, Julian. 1971. "The Inverse Care Law." *The Lancet* 1 (7696): 405–12.

Turkish Daily News. 2003. "Turkish Health Workers Protest Inadequate Funding." November 6.

UNAIDS (Joint United Nations Programme on HIV/AIDS). 2004. *2004 Report on the Global AIDS Epidemic: 4th Global Report*. Geneva.

U.S. Institute of Medicine. 2004. *In the Nation's Compelling Interest: Ensuring Diversity in the Health Care Workforce*. Washington, D.C.: National Academies Press. [Retrieved October 6, 2004, from www.nap.edu/books/ 030909125X/html/]

Van Lerberghe, Wim, Calaudia Conceicao, Wim van Damme, and Paulo Ferrinho. 2002. "When Staff is Underpaid: Dealing with the Individual Coping Strategies of Health Personnel." *Bulletin of the World Health Organization* 80 (7): 581–84.

Van Rensburg, Dingie, and Nicolaas van Rensburg. 1999. "Distribution of Human Resources." In Nicholas Crisp, ed., *South African Health Review 1999*. Durban: Health Systems Trust. [www.hst.org.za/sahr].

Vatankhah, Soudabeh. 2002. "Human Resource Development for Health in the Islamic Republic of Iran." Paper presented at the 49th Session of the WHO Regional Committee for the Eastern Mediterranean, Cairo, October 2002. [Retrieved October 6, 2004, from www.emro.who.int/RC49/RC49-10%20IranPresentation Paper.doc].

Vaz, F., S. Bergstrom, L. Vaz Mda, J. Langa, and A. Bugalho. 1999. "Training Medical Assistants for Surgery." *Bulletin of the World Health Organization* 77 (8): 688–91.

Vlassoff, C., and S. Fonn. 2001. "Health Workers for Change as a Health Systems Management and Development Tool." *Health Policy and Planning* 16 (Suppl 1): 47–52.

Vujicic, M., P. Zurn, K. Diallo, O. Adams, and M. Dal Poz. 2004. "The Role of Wages in the Migration of Health Care Professionals from Developing Countries." *Human Resources for Health* 2 (1): 3.

Wagstaff, Adam, and Marium Claeson. 2004. *The Millennium Development Goals for Health—Rising to the Challenges*. Washington, D.C.: World Bank.

Walker, Liz, and Lucy Gilson. 2004. "'We Are Bitter But We Are Satisfied': Nurses as Street-Level Bureaucrats in South Africa." *Social Science & Medicine* 59 (6): 1251–61.

Wibulpolprasert, Suwit. 1999. "Inequitable Distribution of Doctors: Can It Be Solved?" *Human Resources for Health Development Journal* 3 (1): 2–39.

Wibulpolprasert, Suwit, and Paichit Pengpaibon. 2003. "Integrated Strategies to Tackle Inequitable Distribution of Doctors in Thailand: Four Decades of Experience." *Human Resources for Health* 1(12).

W. K. Kellogg Foundation. Undated. "UNI: Community Partnerships for Health Professions Education. Helping Communities Take Care of Health Care." [Retrieved October 6, 2004, from www.wkkf.org/pubs/Pub3358. pdf].

World Bank. 2003a. "Bolivia: Health Sector Reforms in the Context of Decentralization." Human Development Department, Latin America, and the Caribbean Region,

Report 26140-BO. Washington, D.C.

———. 2003b. *Ghana Poverty Reduction Strategy—An Agenda for Growth and Prosperity, 2003–2005.* Vol. 1: Analysis and Policy Statement. [Retrieved October 6, 2004, from http://siteresources.worldbank.org/GHANAEXTN/Resources/Ghana_PRSP.pdf].

———. 2003c. "Project Appraisal Document on a Proposed Development Credit and Development Grant for a Health Sector Program Support Project II." Human Development II, Africa Regional Office, Report 24842-GH. Washington, D.C.

———. 2004a. *Program Document for a Proposed Credit and Grant to Ghana for a Second Poverty Reduction Support Credit.* Poverty Reduction and Management 4, Africa Region, Report 29177-GH.

———. 2004b. *World Development Report 2004: Making Services Work for Poor People.* Washington, D.C.: Oxford University Press.

WHO (World Health Organization). 2000. *World Directory of Medical Schools*, 7th edition. [Retrieved October 6, 2004, from www.wpro.who.int/applics/medschool/default.cfm].

———. 2002. "Technical Consultation on Imbalances in the Health Workforce." Geneva. [Retrieved October 6, 2004, from www.who.int/hrh/documents/en/consultation_imbalances.pdf].

———. 2004. "WHO Estimates of Health Personnel: Physicians, Nurses, Midwives, Dentists, Pharmacists." Geneva.

WHO-Europe. 2004. *Health for All Database*. Version June 2004. [Retrieved October 6, 2004, from http://hfadb.who.dk/hfa/].

Wyss, Kaspar, N'Diekhor Yemadji, and Christoph Kurowski. 2003. "Besoins et disponibilite des ressources humaines dans le cadre de l'elargissement des systemes de sante en direction des objectifs internationaux de developpement: Le cas du Tchad." Swiss Tropical Institute, Basel.

Youlong, G., A. Wilkes, and G. Bloom. 1997. "Health Human Resource Development in Rural China." *Health Policy and Planning* 12 (4): 320–28.

Zaidi, S. A. 1986. "Why Medical Students Will Not Practice in Rural Areas: Evidence from a Survey." *Social Science and Medicine* 22 (5): 527–33.

Zurn, Pascal, Mario Dal Poz, Barbara Stilwell, and Orvill Adams. 2002. "Imbalances in the Health Workforce." Briefing Paper. World Health Organization, Geneva.

3

Global
responsibilities

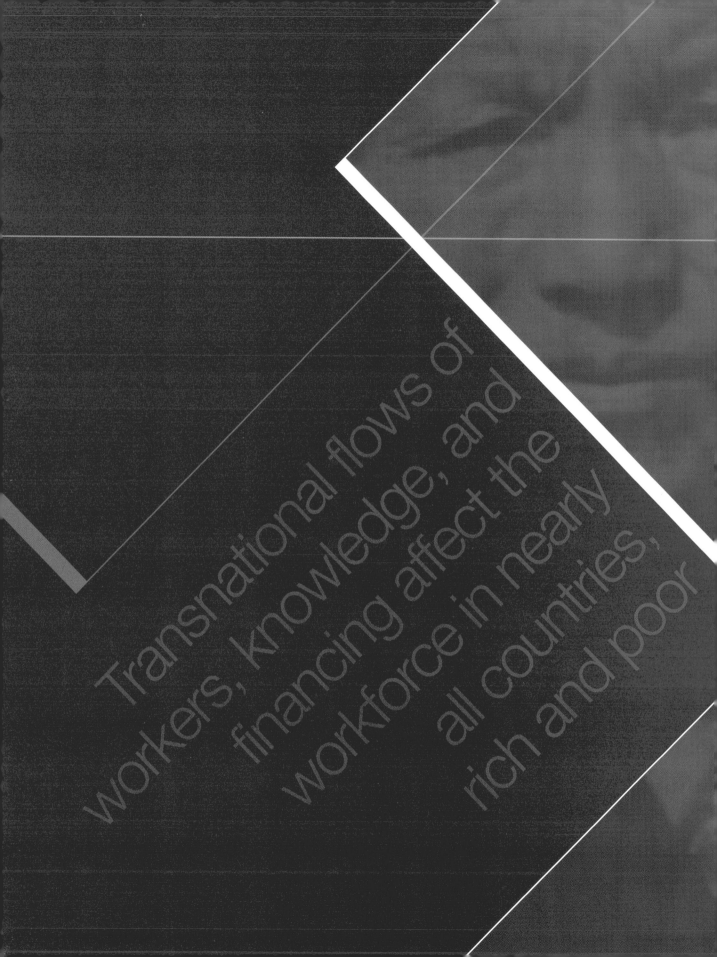

Transnational flows of workers, knowledge, and financing affect the workforce in nearly all countries, rich and poor

Global Responsibilities

No country can fully control all aspects of its workforce development. Transnational flows of workers, knowledge, and financing affect the workforce in nearly all countries, rich and poor. And in today's globalizing world, these cross-border flows are accelerating—with uncertain and complex consequences, benefiting some, increasing the vulnerability of others. Stakeholders at the national, regional, and global levels—governments, agencies, academia, civil society—all confront the challenge of taking advantage of these flows for advancing national and global health. Managing better these global flows is absolutely critical for supporting the country-led strategies presented in chapter 3.

Left unattended, transnational flows can have serious, even catastrophic effects, on national and local efforts. But properly harnessed, they have great potential for advancing equitable global health and development. The international spread of infectious diseases—such as HIV/AIDS, the recent SARS and highly pathogenic Asian flu epidemics—challenges international actors to mount a unified defense against lethal pathogens. Although potentially devastating, the new threats prompt stronger and faster sharing of knowledge and technologies to control lethal pathogens. And the devastating effect of AIDS on the workforce in sub-Saharan Africa and the push for the rapid scaling up of interventions to combat HIV/AIDS, tuberculosis, and malaria have brought to the fore the urgent need to strengthen weak health systems and particularly the workforce to deliver essential interventions. In this context the "brain drain" of skilled workers from low-income to high-income countries is particularly alarming.

This chapter presents a strategic approach to managing three flows that influence workforce

❝❝ Of various migration streams, the most controversial is that of highly skilled medical professionals from poorer southern to richer northern countries

performance—worker migration, the dissemination of knowledge, and overseas development assistance.

Migration: Fatal flows

In search of a better life, millions of health workers decide where to work and for whom. In every community, region, and nation, employers and workers seek each other out to make arrangements for conducting work. These labor markets have become more global, and with shortages in many high-income countries, the choices available to sought-after workers are expanding.

Most migration of health workers is within countries. Health workers typically move from rural areas to urban centers, and most countries have an urban concentration of professionals. Migration can also be quite extensive among neighboring countries. Movements of medical professionals, for example, are well established among neighboring countries in the Southern African and North American regions. In general, the gradient is from inferior to superior work and more stable political and economically rewarding situations. The movements are not unidirectional, however—they are in many directions, resembling a "carousel effect."[1] Nor is it only the workers who move. Patients can move to providers abroad, and medical services (x-ray diagnostics) can be delivered electronically.

Of various migration streams, the most controversial is that of highly skilled professionals from poorer southern to richer northern countries, mostly doctors and nurses with equivalency certification in source and destination countries. Dentists, pharmacists, and technicians are also in global demand. These movements add to the already severe workforce imbalances described

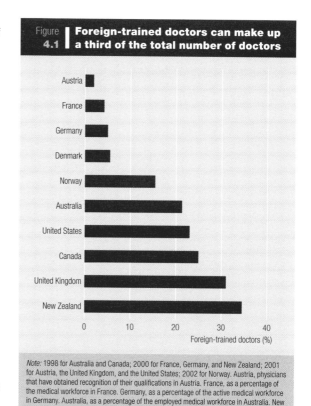

Figure 4.1 | **Foreign-trained doctors can make up a third of the total number of doctors**

Note: 1998 for Australia and Canada; 2000 for France, Germany, and New Zealand; 2001 for Austria, the United Kingdom, and the United States; 2002 for Norway. Austria, physicians that have obtained recognition of their qualifications in Austria. France, as a percentage of the medical workforce in France. Germany, as a percentage of the active medical workforce in Germany. Australia, as a percentage of the employed medical workforce in Australia. New Zealand, as a percentage of the active medical practioners in New Zealand.
Source: OECD 2002.

in chapter 1. They compromise the capacity of health systems in source countries. And they are tantamount to a massive subsidy from the poor to the rich. With the cost of training a general practice doctor estimated at $60,000 and that of training other medical auxiliaries $12,000, the African Union estimates that low-income countries subsidize high-income countries with $500 million a year through the movement of health workers.[2]

Statistical data are fragmentary, but administrative data pieced together from professional certifications provide a snapshot of global migration patterns. Most source countries are in Africa, the Caribbean,

> **Many, if not most, northern importing countries are chronically dependent on southern countries for a significant share of their nurses and doctors**

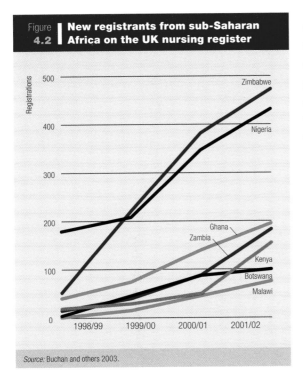

Figure 4.2 New registrants from sub-Saharan Africa on the UK nursing register

Source: Buchan and others 2003.

Southeast Asia, and South Asia, with their workers moving to such destination countries as Australia, Canada, France, Belgium, the United Kingdom, and the United States. Confirming these flows are the high proportions of foreign-trained professionals in northern countries, up to a third of the workforce (figure 4.1).[3] There is also suggestive evidence of accelerating migration—especially for nurses in the past decade. Consider the upsurge of African-trained nurses registering for work in the United Kingdom in the latter half of the 1990s (figure 4.2).

Migration patterns are generated by "push" and "pull" factors along channels facilitated by labor markets, linguistic compatibility, sociocultural affinity, professional equivalency, and visa policies. Six factors have been proposed as driving these movements: income, job satisfaction, career opportunity, governance and management, safety and risks, and social and family reasons.[4] The pattern of South Africa importing workers from Cuba and neighboring African countries while exporting workers to wealthier Anglophone countries illustrates the complexity of these movements (figure 4.3).

Many, if not most, northern importing countries are chronically dependent on southern countries for a significant share of their nurses and doctors— because of domestic under-production, aging populations, advancing technology, changing family structures, and rising consumer demand. The current stock of nurses in the United States, already in shortage, is predicted to fall below 20 percent of projected workforce requirements by 2020.[5] In Eastern Europe economic and political transitions are leading to the restructuring of health systems, with a realignment of health workers. With wages several-fold higher in the West, major migration streams are likely to develop between Eastern and Western Europe with the expansion of the European Union.[6]

Southern exporting countries are of two types: strategic exporters whose out-migration is policy-supported, and unwilling exporters, whose migratory streams are not supported by national health policy. The former include Cuba, India, Egypt, and the Philippines, which purposefully export workers, including medical personnel, to gain skills, earn foreign exchange, or fulfill humanitarian aims. The latter include many countries in Africa, the Caribbean, and Asia, where out-migration is driven by global labor market forces against the intent of national health policies. In some of these countries, ministries of finance and planning may not support the concerns of health ministries over the loss of health workers.

> ❝ **People on the losing end are those whose well-being depends on access to health services and where out-migration aggravates human resource shortages**

Figure 4.3 | **South Africa: Main channels for out and in-migration**

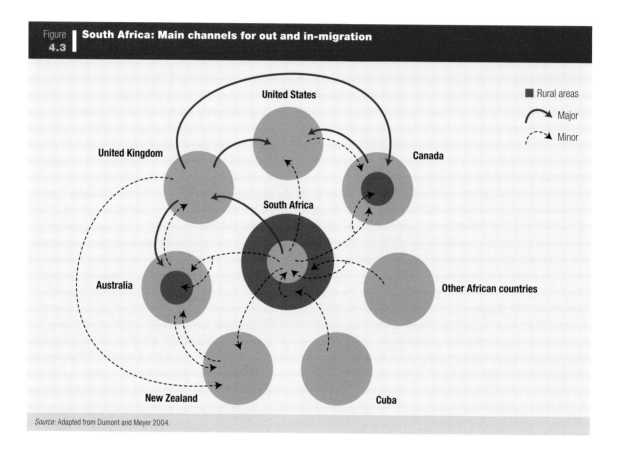

■ Rural areas

↷➤ Major

⤏➤ Minor

Source: Adapted from Dumont and Meyer 2004.

Who are the winners in medical migration? Migrants are able to improve their compensation and career opportunities, while also better supporting their families, including extended members, in their home country. Wealthier destination countries can bridge their workforce gaps and adequately staff their medical institutions—especially the public facilities in remote regions that commonly fail to attract domestic workers.

People on the losing end are those whose well-being depends on access to health services and where out-migration aggravates human resource shortages. There is little doubt that well-trained

professionals are vital for education, training, research and development, advanced specialized care, secondary care, staff supervision, and technical guidance. While the absolute numbers may not be large, the outflows can be "fatal" for disadvantaged people in source countries.

In 2001, 382 nurses migrated from Zimbabwe to the United Kingdom.[7] This increased the United Kingdom nursing stock by only 0.1 percent but the loss to Zimbabwe's nursing stock was 40 times greater in percentage terms. Migration can also affect key services or regions. Wholesale recruitment of the nursing staff of an intensive care

> **Strategies must be crafted to channel, balance, and manage migration to provide good and equitable global health while mitigating harm in both source and destination countries**

unit at a Filipino hospital essentially closed those services to the local population.[8] The migration of service workers from Malawi to the United Kingdom is leading to the near collapse of maternity service workers in Malawi's central hospital.[9]

The exodus is often only the beginning of a downward spiral of health system capacity. In health facilities already facing shortages of staff and unfilled vacancies, the migration of existing staff adds to the workload of workers who remain, increasing their case loads and over time, leading to fatigue, a loss of motivation, and eventual burnout. These pressures provide an impetus for remaining workers to themselves migrate out—perpetuating the vicious spiral. The loss of workers also results in leakages of public subsidies invested in educating them.

How, then, to deal with international migration? At one extreme are those who argue that medical migration from poor to rich countries should be stopped. The health consequences of the hemorrhaging of skilled professionals from source countries are catastrophic. The poaching of highly capable human resources is predatory behavior, unethical and deleterious to health. At the other extreme are those who defend the basic human right of professionals to move. An open international labor market offers efficiency and economic gains. Diasporas also generate remittances and create a brain gain and brain circulation, rather than a brain drain, by sending back ideas, entrepreneurship, and technology. The free movement of labor also advances global economic equity.

Neither extreme produces viable strategies. Blocking worker flows violates human rights and is unenforceable. Leaving migration to labor markets turns a blind eye to "fatal flows." Instead,

strategies must be crafted to channel, balance, and manage migration to provide good and equitable global health while mitigating harm in both source and destination countries. In so doing, the disproportionate power of richer countries to control migration streams should be recognized.

A set of balanced strategies would concentrate on retaining talent in source countries, attaining self-sufficiency in destination countries, and expanding global opportunities.

Retaining talent
To address the out-migration of highly skilled professionals, source countries may pursue both protective and corrective strategies. Protective strategies attempt to retain workers, slowing out-migration. Corrective strategies invest in the production of health workers to meet national requirements and exploit international demand.

To dampen push forces for out-migration, protective strategies should address the determinants of "motivation"—achieving satisfactory remuneration, creating positive work environments, and developing supportive systems (chapter 3). Improving wages alone is unlikely to be enough given the huge salary differences between source and destination countries. But much more can be done, within fiscal constraints, in work environments, nonfinancial incentives, management practices, and systems support.[10]

Workers frequently complain about professional factors that shape career development.[11] They also express dissatisfaction with management malpractices—poor leadership and little autonomy, support, recognition, or team work. The poor synchronization of drugs and supplies as well as concerns about physical insecurity and safety are

> **" Corrective strategies can capitalize on the abundance of potential human capital in low-income countries by ramping up training and educational investments**

symptomatic of weak systems support. Recognizing these internal problems, the New Partnership for Africa's Development (NEPAD) has called for the creation of "necessary political, social, and economic conditions that would serve as incentives to curb the brain drain."[12] Development partners can help stem migration by investing in conditions that foster retention.

Another protective strategy is to erect barriers to out-migration. Frequently instituted is bonding graduates by directing them to national rural service after graduation. Other bonding schemes call for reimbursing the cost of public education or making candidates ineligible for specialty training if they do not fulfill mandatory in-country service. Attempts can also be made to restrict travel, control passports, or impose income taxes on citizens abroad.[13] But enforcing these barriers is very difficult, if not impossible.[14]

Corrective strategies, by recognizing the growing demand for workers, can capitalize on the abundance of potential human capital in low-income countries by ramping up training and educational investments. In some countries the very heavy loss of highly skilled professionals presents an opportunity to restructure the national workforce dramatically—perhaps through massive mobilization, training, and deployment of new cadres of auxiliaries. Recruitment would focus on workers from local communities, and training would offer instruction in local languages and curricula tailored to national, not international, priorities.

In its recent health sector development plan, Ethiopia proposes to train tens of thousands of female school leavers as community health workers, with only locally recognized credentials. Professional councils that resist the delegation of skills to auxiliaries may be persuaded to relax rigid regulations, many inherited from colonial regimes.[15] With heavy out-migration, these councils face the diminishing political clout of their dwindling numbers, while having to respond to health crises.

Career planning is just as important for auxiliaries as for highly trained professionals. The lack of career prospects can demotivate workers, irrespective of level. The frustration of mother-and-child aides in Tanzania was one factor in the government's stopping the training of aides and upgrading their skills and certification to nurses (making them mobile internationally).[16]

Attaining self-sufficiency

In the competition for scarce health professionals, high-income countries have enormous power to induce inflow of workers from low-income countries. And because they benefit from international migration, there is little incentive for them to change policy. After all, imports enable these countries to quickly meet their requirements without financial and institutional investments. Yet, it would be wise for rich countries to strive for self-sufficiency, because reliance on international recruitment is short-sighted, inequitable, and risky. Building a pipeline to produce highly skilled personnel is both sound and fair.

In most high-income countries, the demand for health services and health personnel has been growing much faster than supply, and the resulting shortages are likely to worsen. In large part, this is due to aging populations in rich countries, which are consuming more health care services. In Canada, the supply of physicians and nurses—given production, out-migration, and attrition—is not expected to keep pace with population growth over the next two decades.[17] Australia reports a lack of 5,000 nurses;

> **A global educational reinvestment fund would be a win-win approach to international migration, intensifying investments in educational capacity in source countries**

a recent survey in the United States indicated as many as 126,000 nurse positions are waiting to be filled.[18] Each of these shortages is projected to grow many times over the next several decades.[19]

To get more health workers, private and public groups in rich countries recruit them from overseas.[20] Concerns about misuse and abuse in recruitment have led governments and agencies to formulate codes of practice, encouraging self-policing among countries that actively recruit health workers. For example, destination countries should not recruit from countries with severe human resource shortages. Similarly, a quota or cap of visas might be imposed on professional migrants from distressed countries. Most of these codes are just being implemented, so their impact is yet to be determined.[21] Systematic experience with these codes could eventually develop into a global system to promote and enforce a universal code on ethical recruitment (box 4.1).

Expanding global opportunities

Besides individual country action, new opportunities are opening for global regimes to manage migration for mutual health benefits: creating an educational reinvestment fund, accelerating reverse flows, and developing new policies in the global trade of health services. These opportunities are being examined by a new Global Commission on International Migration (box 4.2).

Educational reinvestment fund. A global educational reinvestment fund would be a win-win approach to international migration, intensifying investments in educational capacity in source countries. Given the huge global shortages, the fund would accelerate the development of talent in poorer countries,

---

Box 4.1 | Codes of practice on international recruitment

With the international migration of health professionals hurting many low-income countries, codes of practice are being developed on ethical recruitment. These codes typically have three objectives: protecting individuals in recruitment and employment, ensuring individuals are properly prepared and supported in the job, and protecting countries from unethical and aggressive recruitment.

The process of developing the codes has greatly raised awareness of their potential impact on health care systems elsewhere. Their use could be strengthened by:

- Learning from the "early adopters."
- Focusing on protecting the health systems of other countries.
- Strengthening the systems for implementation— particularly for monitoring compliance and using incentives and sanctions.
- For the global codes, using incentives and sanctions may be more difficult and could be replaced by producing better data in countries losing staff, showing the numbers and destinations of their emigrants.
- Exerting external pressure, such as that from civil society organizations, to ensure that the codes are being followed.

Source: Willetts and Martineau 2004.

---

supporting public efforts and offering incentives for private investments. Training would enjoy the advantage of lower unit costs and new institutional arrangements. Regional collaborations among academic institutions, including credit-sharing, could strengthen existing training programs and promote access for individuals in countries not yet able to support their own educational programs. Investments in improving managerial capacity in education and

Box
4.2 | **The Global Commission on International Migration**

The Global Commission on International Migration, co-chaired by Mamphela Ramphele and Jan Karlsson, was endorsed by the UN Secretary-General and launched in December 2003. The Commission is developing a framework for a coherent and comprehensive global response to migration challenges. With about 175 million migrants worldwide, the phenomenon of international migration impacts all countries and sectors of employment. A combination of global trends in demographics, economics, conflict and insecurity, travel and communications has created powerful forces for movement across borders.

Among the areas of concern for the commission are three issues that have direct implications for global human resources for health.

- The first is "migrants in the global labor market." The Commission hopes to shed light on emerging labor market scenarios and the various options for policymakers and other stakeholders.
- Second is "migration, development, and poverty reduction." The Commission will examine the policy implications of brain drain, brain gain, and brain circulation. It will also address the impact of migrant

remittances, return migration, and assisted reintegration.

- Third is "migrants in society." This research will cover the policy challenges related to the social and cultural dimensions of international migration. Topics will include migrant rights, citizenship, host societies and culture, integration, and the role of family reunions and social networks as drivers for migration.

The Commission is set to issue a final report in the summer of 2005. Its recommendations will guide national and international policymaking on the retention and migration of health professionals.

Source: Global Commission on International Migration, [www.gcim.org].

training in source countries could also be intensified. The fund should support public efforts while offering incentives for private investments in education.

The fund would not offer compensation for migration losses. Attempts to develop strict compensatory payment are unlikely to be successful.[22] A reimbursement mechanism would require impossibly close monitoring of worker movements to determine the size of compensation. Who should provide and receive the compensation is not clear cut and computing forgone educational investments is not straightforward. How would public versus private investment be accounted for? Most important, the requisite political commitment is not forthcoming. Without political support, neither a voluntary nor a compulsory fund is feasible.

Why, then, should rich countries contribute to a voluntary educational reinvestment fund? First, the evidence is clear that the financial loss to source countries is significant. In India, the cost of training physicians is as high as 70 times the per capita GDP.[23] The South African Department of Health estimates the cost of training a physician at 23 times the GDP per capita, and that of the training a nurse at 10 times.[24] Based on South African migration statistics, the department estimates forgone investment of around $1 billion, equivalent to 17 percent of national public health spending in 2000.

Second, political commitment to the Millennium Development Goals argues strongly for making such cost-effective investments. The fund would help advance health and educational targets. Third,

❝❞ Another global strategy is to flip migration from a one-way process of brain drain to promote appropriate 'reverse flows'

political pressures and public embarrassment are likely to grow as workforce shortages in the midst of health crises become linked to rich country poaching of medical workers from these source countries. The patently unfair practices with devastating health consequences—the fatal flows—are likely to grow in political and public debate. A voluntary contributory educational investment fund would be a sensible way of addressing the stark imbalances.

Reversing flows. Another global strategy is to flip migration from a one-way process of brain drain to promote appropriate "reverse flows" in a more dynamic multidirectional process of brain circulation and gain. Countries importing medical personnel can step up their exports, and diaspora communities could accelerate two-way flows. Fresh proposals are emerging for volunteer cadres, expansion of nongovernmental activities, and north-south twinning or partnership arrangements.

Exporting countries—Cuba, Egypt, India, and the Philippines—could accelerate their flows to severe shortage countries. Indeed, Cuba already provides significant human resources to many African and Caribbean nations (box 4.3). India reportedly has accelerated its training programs for doctors and nurses, many by the private sector for export to anglophone countries. Egyptian professionals offer their services throughout the Arabic-speaking world. Note, however, that except for Cuba, exporting countries mainly aim at richer OECD countries. The sending countries also suffer simultaneously from internal maldistributions. India and the Philippines export to overseas markets while leaving staff posts vacant in deprived regions (box 4.4).

The diaspora need not be seen as a permanent national loss, for health workers in diaspora communities can offer remittances, skills, and contacts.[25] Over the past decade, total international remittances have more than doubled from $33 billion in 1992 to $80 billion by 2002, now constituting the second largest flow of external funds to developing countries.[26] These remittances have also become a source of investment capital in the health sector.[27] And overseas health workers could be encouraged to return—permanently or temporarily.

Ironically, severely worker-deficient countries sometimes have the most stringent immigration laws and restrictive licensing and registration systems for foreigners. The IOM's Reintegration Programme of Qualified African Nationals has relocated only 2,000 nationals to 11 source countries in 15 years. Others are experimenting with tapping knowledge and skills of professionals abroad.[28] More than 80 diaspora groups are experimenting with knowledge networks, including the Retransfer of Technology to Turkey initiative of the UNDP and the Virtual Laboratory Toolkit of UNESCO.

New reverse flows are also on the rise. International and faith-based nongovernmental organizations are dispatching more foreign health workers to severely worker-deficient countries. A variety of south-north twinning and partnership arrangements are being proposed and developed. A recent report by the Institute of Medicine in the United States recommended an "AIDSCorp" to address the human resource bottleneck in tackling HIV/AIDS treatment and prevention.[29] One innovative possibility is recruiting health workers from displaced refugees who might otherwise linger in camps for years.

❝ **Creating win-win situations for source and destination countries should be a priority for a global mobility regime**

Box 4.3 | Cuba's international health workforce

Since 1960 more than 67,000 Cuban health professionals have served in public health roles in 94 countries, and more than 9,000 students from 83 countries have been enrolled in Cuban medical education institutions.

The first Cuban medical team was sent to earthquake devastated Chile in 1960, when the two governments had no formal relations. Such disaster relief missions were dispatched to another 16 countries over the next decades. But Cuban health professionals—the vast majority of them physicians—also began serving Asia, Africa, and Latin America and the Caribbean.

Since the 1963 request from Algeria—then bereft of physicians at the end of French occupation—another 92 governments have initiated pacts with Cuba for a sustained presence of Cuban health professionals in their countries' health care delivery programs.

Half this cooperation began in the 1990s, speaking to developments in Cuba's own health system. By mid-decade, the neighborhood-based family doctor-and-nurse

program was in place across the country, and by 1999 it covered 98 percent of Cuba's 11 million people. The program was the culmination of a process of embedding health services deeper into communities, aimed at more effective health promotion and disease prevention. Curricula in Cuba's 22 medical schools were revamped, and a three-year residency in family medicine ratcheted up the annual number of graduates. By the end of the decade, Cuba had nearly 30,000 family physicians and some 60,000 doctors (70,000 by the 2004 graduation, more than sub-Saharan Africa).

In 1998 hurricanes George and Mitch swept through Central America and the Caribbean, leaving 2.4 million homeless. Cuban medical teams, first deployed on an emergency basis, stayed on at the request of several governments under Cuba's Comprehensive Health Program, created in response to the region's crisis and later expanded to include a total of 22 countries in Latin America, the Caribbean, Africa, and Asia. By the end of 2003, there were 530 Cuban health professionals

in Guatemala, 578 in Haiti, 113 in Belize, 262 in Honduras,122 in Botswana, 178 in Ghana, 107 in Mali, and 231 in The Gambia.

Under these agreements, the host country provides accommodations and food, domestic transportation, a place of work, and a monthly stipend (usually $100), while Cuban personnel receive their regular salaries, airfare, and other logistical support from the Cuban health ministry. In other arrangements with wealthier countries such as South Africa, the host government pays additional salary, part kept by the professionals and part remitted to the Cuban health ministry.

Recently, Cuba has initiated trilateral collaboration, with a third country or agency donating resources for health programs. For the 2001–02 vaccination drive in Haiti, Cuban epidemiologists and family doctors teamed up with Haitian health authorities to immunize 800,000 children against five childhood diseases. Funds from the French government and 2 million doses of vaccines from the Japanese government completed the triangle.

Source: Ministry of Public Health 2003a, 2003c, 2004a, 2004b; Ministry of Foreign Relations and the Vice Ministry for Medical Education 2004; Maamar 2003; Reed 2000; Castro 2003; Bourne and Reed 2003a.

Medical tourists. Patients also move to service providers, and some services, such as radiology and diagnostics, can be transmitted over new information and communications pathways.

Thailand, Singapore, and some Gulf states have deliberately cultivated their domestic specialized health infrastructure to attract "medical tourists" from abroad. In these cases, the temporary migrants are

> **Patients can also move to service providers, and some services can be transmitted over new information and communication pathways**

Box 4.4 | Health worker migration: A global phenomenon

Medical migration affects all world regions. Most oil-exporting societies import health workers from such countries as Egypt, India, and the Philippines. The Caribbean is a major source of health workers for North America. Western Europe is increasingly attracting workers from eastern Europe.

Among these countries, the Philippines is one of the world's leading exporters of nurses. Importing countries are particularly attracted to the English-speaking talent, and in 2003 an estimated 25,000 nurses left the Philippines to such countries as the United Kingdom, Saudi Arabia, Canada, and the United States—three times the number graduating from nursing school.

For many, this is a win-win situation. Importing countries solve their workforce shortage

problems quickly, with little need for investment in salaries or in domestic recruitment and training campaigns. Filipino nurses are able to earn as much as 20 times what they would earn in the Philippines, contributing to improving the quality of life of their families.

Yet the benefits of nurse out-migration from the Philippines can be offset by unintended

consequences. Entire nursing units are migrating, leaving hospitals wholly understaffed. Filipino doctors—as well as pharmacists, physical therapists, dentists, orderlies, and even engineers and teachers—are retraining as nurses to be able to capitalize on lucrative foreign nursing positions, further threatening the health care system and the general economy.

Nurses leaving the Philippines

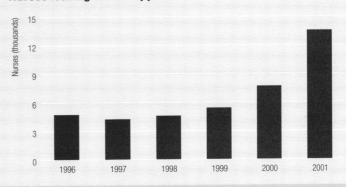

Source: BBC News 2002, 2003a, 2003b; San Francisco Chronicle 2003; Chan 2003; WHO 2003; Washington Post Foreign Service 2004.

patients rather than departing medical professionals. In Thailand meeting the demands of "medical tourism" is estimated to absorb 15 percent of the highly skilled medical personnel in the country.[30] Another flow is remote diagnostic services, such as x-rays and electrocardiogram readings.

Liberalizing trade in medical personnel. Creating win-win situations for source and destination countries should be a priority for the World Trade Organization (WTO) in trade liberalization negotiations under

mode 4 of the General Agreement on Trade and Services (GATS). Few countries are yet committed to a serious liberalization of the trade of medical personnel.[31] But several high-income countries facing significant health worker shortages have introduced provisions in their immigration legislation to facilitate the entry of certain categories of medical personnel. Others are likely to follow. Because there is no substitute for skilled medical labor, powerful lobbies will continue to push governments for further liberalization of trade under mode 4 in future rounds

❝ **The transfer of knowledge on effective interventions can improve health everywhere—especially among the poor**

of negotiations.[32] Balancing these pressures with the needs of worker-deficient low-income countries will be a major challenge for WTO members.

Knowledge: An under-tapped resource

Health services are based on knowledge—the knowledge of health workers—not only of science-related inputs (drugs and vaccines) but also of information and analyses that inform and guide social action. Knowledge spans a wide range of themes—data and metrics, appraisal tools, analyses and research, standards and best practices. It is local as well as global, and implicit as well as explicit. Local solutions depend upon local knowledge that contributes to, and is adaptable from, global knowledge. Explicit knowledge is consolidated in books and journals, while the "know-how" of implicit knowledge comes from human experience.

The application of knowledge to develop new interventions and its transfer can improve health everywhere—but particularly among the poor. The discovery of germ theory provided the foundation for the control of infectious diseases. New vaccines and drugs offered unprecedented preventive and therapeutic powers. Epidemiologic methods made it possible to asses risk factors for disease and the effectiveness of clinical interventions. While much of this knowledge was biomedical and thus easily transferable across populations, equally important social, economic, and managerial knowledge, as well as traditional and indigenous knowledge, was also accumulated, improving the performance of public and clinical health services.

The international diffusion of knowledge can support national efforts—powerfully. The remarkable convergence of health between the world's poorest and richest societies over the 20th century has been attributed to this diffusion.[33] At the beginning of the century, rich and poor countries had gaps in average longevity of about four decades. By the end of the century, the gap had narrowed to about two decades. Without the HIV/AIDS epidemic interrupting this century-old trend, the convergence could have carried forward well into this century.

Although knowledge has enormous potential to improve workforce policies and management, it remains an underused resource. Knowledge of the functioning of health systems and the provision of health services is lagging. Only recently have human resources become the focus of systematic data collection and analyses.[34] The knowledge of how to improve the performance of health workers is particularly inadequate: it is underproduced, poorly disseminated, and insufficiently applied.

Accurate data about the numbers of health workers—including community health workers, traditional healers, and auxiliary workers—are essential for country-level decisionmaking, as are workforce statistics on gender, age structure, ethnicity, educational attainment, geographical distribution, public-private sector distribution, unemployment, and migration. Yet some ministries of health lack even basic information on the number, type, and location of the national workforce. And available tools and methods for planning and management are not yet well adapted to help plan and manage complex and rapidly changing workforce dynamics.

Strategic planning of human investments requires local information backed by globally validated knowledge and tools to appraise the situation and design future investments. Adopting "good practices" learned in diverse settings around the world strengthens management. Results-based monitoring and evaluation systems guide continuous improvements. In every country, the migration of workers affects numeric adequacy and geographic distribution, just as the work environment influences migration decisions. Especially in health crisis countries, the financing of the workforce is inextricably linked to foreign aid flows. Understanding and managing international flows can help strengthen national programs while building the foundation for collective global action.

Yet, as a technical field, human resources has few communities of knowledge creation, sharing, and practice. In this comparatively neglected field, research has not been robust. Few research units or institutions specialize in human resources for health. Of great practical importance is the lack of a center of gravity of technical capabilities and assistance in workforce policy and management. Technical institutions in low-income countries are grossly under-financed and thus unable to generate a critical technical mass. Technical institutions in high-income countries enjoy better funding, but much of their work is irrelevant to the challenges of low-income countries. The WHO collates global statistics on the workforce, but most international agencies are bereft of core technical expertise in this underfinanced field.

The potential to harness knowledge for improved workforce policy and management is great—even modest efforts could enhance the impact of existing knowledge on practical application. Three strategies should be pursued to mobilize the power of knowledge: bridging the knowledge-action gap, sharing information and knowledge, and strengthening the knowledge base.

Bridging the knowledge-action gap

Bridging the "know-do gap"—the distance between knowledge and practice, between knowing what to do, knowing how to do it, and doing it—is a key priority.[35] More than research it requires better application of what we already know. Nearly half the world's deaths are theoretically preventable with available knowledge, technologies, and resources. The failure is the inability of our health systems to make knowledge and technologies available to people who need them.

The lag time from knowledge generation to its application, often far too long, should be reduced. For instance, for innovative health care practices in the United States, the lag has been estimated at 15–20 years.[36] This could be shortened by establishing much stronger links between the provision of health services and research geared to tackling problems that hamper the delivery of health interventions. Learning from research on the downstream impacts of HIV/AIDS on rural communities in Africa has had a similar 15–20 year lag.[37] Starting with action stimulates the mobilization of available knowledge, sparking an action-learning cycle of information accrual, stocktaking, appraisal, and translating lessons into action to improve performance.

Good health information can guide effective action. An ideal health information system should track data on:

- Health outcomes (mortality, morbidity, diseases, and health status).
- Health system performance (service availability, quality, use, and coverage).
- Health system inputs (infrastructure, drugs, equipment, human and financial resources).

These data should be organized by key stratifiers, such as gender, socioeconomic status, geography, and ethnicity.[38]

4

GLOBAL RESPONSIBILITIES

" The pace and depth of global learning will depend on the commitment to work and learn together across boundaries

Such data are rarely available in the countries that need readily applicable information the most. Even simple head counts would help clarify the workforce situations and enable programs to set goals and track progress. Irrespective of current weaknesses, every country should mobilize whatever data are currently available. In time, the database can be improved, including information on workforce increments, attrition, and health labor market outcomes. International standards for information systems supplemented with technical assistance should be developed to strengthen national efforts by improving the quality and relevance of data—and harmonizing data for cross-national analyses.

More than a dozen appraisal instruments have been developed to help decisionmakers obtain a clear picture for planning and management (box 4.5). The earliest were developed for manpower planning. Some of the latest tackle workforce planning for HIV/AIDS prevention and treatment. And some have been simplified in computer-based programs to enhance user-friendliness.

The current set of instruments is adequate for starting country work, though their validity, usefulness, and robustness need to be strengthened. And supplemental instruments—political mapping of stakeholders, costing exercises to determine financial requirements, promotion and regulation of the private sector, and checklists of medical regulations—should fortify the toolkit. The tools should be tested, applied, and validated in country situations, with field experience contributing to global learning for a core set of instruments to guide national action.

Sharing information and knowledge
Some sharing of knowledge is in the marketplace, associated with commercial activities, and some

is in communities of practice. The pace and depth of global learning on human resources for health will depend on the commitment to work and learn together across boundaries. The Health Metrics Network is developing one such learning system in health information. The human resource observatory in the Americas is another example of regional collaboration to link communities of practice to share knowledge (box 4.6).

Institutional arrangements and best practice guidelines to train and improve skills of the health workforce are much less developed than they are on other aspects of health. There are few centers of gravity of technical capacity that practitioners can tap into and advance the global knowledge bank. Documentation centers that gather, organize, archive, and disseminate information, ideas, and approaches would fill an important niche. Such centers could be constructed by adding human resource specialization to centers of health systems or health economics and financing. Also useful would be systems for bringing technical practitioners together for pooling experiences, developing codes of application, and strengthening best practices.

Appreciated far too little is the vast experiential base of almost all public health workers in disease control and health systems that craft day-after-day human resource solutions. But these experiences are not being consolidated through technical learning processes. Focal centers of technical capabilities, perhaps linked in a virtual network, could assemble professional teams to address specific technical challenges—assisting countries, poor and rich alike, in grappling with workforce challenges.

The WHO could draw together high quality technical expertise to codify practice standards for

GLOBAL RESPONSIBILITIES

4

114

Box
4.5

Toolkits for appraising health workforces

A proper appraisal of human resource for health needs to be carried out to guide planning, policy, and management. Most appraisals include an assessment of the current workforce and future requirements, including the aims of quality, equity, and efficiency. Where conventional health service providers are in short supply, an analysis of alternative providers might be necessary. And to ensure sustainable solutions, human resource policymaking and systems should be analyzed. A broader understanding of organisational goals, and strengths and weaknesses in areas other than staffing will assist with the development of appropriate and feasible human resource solutions. In addition, an analysis of the policy environment covering stakeholders, opportunities, and threats is needed. The appraisal should identify whether the wider oversight system ensures that human resources are addressed adequately in the health sector.

The JLI conducted a survey of methods and tools currently available for appraising the human resource situation. More than 25 examples of published, unpublished, and web-based materials have been identified. These instruments have been reviewed to identify the purpose and scope, the timeframe, and data requirements. Evidence of their validity has also been sought.

Here's a selection of the instruments:

Instrument	Description	Comments
Broad diagnostic tools		
Human resources in the health sector: guidelines for appraisal and strategic development[a]	Broad analysis of HR situation including HR functions, key stakeholders and policy context. Suggested questions provided.	Also available in French. Information on usage not known.
Reviewing health manpower development: a method of improving national health systems[b]	Explains key issues in areas of HR planning, production and management, sample questions and possible data sources.	Case studies included as examples of the review; may need updating.
Guidelines for a HRH review[c]	Outline a method for making a review and provide suggestions and template materials that can help with data collection and analysis, and with the presentation of the results.	Information on usage not known.
HR planning tools		
Simulation models for workforce planning[d]	Computer-based HR planning model capable of sophisticated projections; much training has been provided for users.	In use for over 10 years and applied on a trial basis in at least eight countries. Also available in Spanish and French.
The WPRO/RTC health workforce planning workbook[e]	Provides steps for developing an HR plan; includes simple computer-based planning model.	Extensively used.
HR management tools		
Achieving the right balance: the role of policy-making processes in managing human resources for health problems[f]	Although designed as study, this contains a framework for analyzing HR policy implementation.	Used for 18 countries; methodology provided, so could be adapted as an assessment tool.
Human resource management assessment instrument for NGOs and public sector health organizations[g]	A rapid tool to assess the core functions of a human resource management system. The tool is adapted to be responsive to HR elements resulting from the impact of HIV/AIDS.	Widely used in both the public and private sectors.
Program-specific HR tools		
Capacity building for 3 by 5: country fact, planning & monitoring sheet[h]	Pro forma to identify current and potential workforce for delivering ART with guidance on information sources.	Supports the WHO ART programme; currently in use.
Human capital development inquiry (for HIV/AIDS programs)[i]	Inquiry to ensure a comprehensive response to entrenched HR issues. Inquiry includes 4 components: policy; HRM; leadership and partnerships.	Still in introductory stage, but useful as a framework to identify range of HR issues to be included in a sustainable strategy.
Tools for considering policy context and options		
Open systems model for institutional appraisal[j]	Situates HR issues in wider organisational context of strategy, culture, management systems, structure, environment, etc.	Would ensure that HR is not forgotten in a broad appraisal exercise.
Decentralization mapping tool[k]	To map out the movement of management responsibilities, including those of human resource management.	An example of a tool for examining the impact of structural reforms; available in Spanish.

Because no single tool covers all the areas to be appraised, a guide is needed to show how existing instruments could be best used to ensure optimal application. And the development and dissemination of more case studies are needed to show how human resource appraisals have been done.

a. Martineau and Martínez 1997. b. Fülöp and Roemer 1987. c. Hall 2001a . d. Hall 2001b. e. Dewdney 2001. f. Egger and others 2000. g. O'Neill 2001. h. WHO undated. i. Management Sciences for Health 2003. j. Department for International Development 2003. k. Management Sciences for Health 2000.
Source: Tim Martineau, Liverpool School of Tropical Medicine, United Kingdom.

4

GLOBAL RESPONSIBILITIES

> **A stronger knowledge base on human resources requires data collection, analysis, and research**

| Box 4.6 | **The PAHO Observatory of Human Resources in Health** |

In 1999 the Pan American Health Organization created the Observatory of Human Resources in Health to respond to the deep and varied human resource challenges facing its 21 member countries. Health authorities, major universities, and professional associations monitor trends in human resource policies, build a consensus around key interventions, and harmonize interests and population needs. Policy analysis and decisions are founded on a core data set consisting of quality of labor and labor regimes, professional education and training for the health workforce, productivity and quality of services, and governance and labor disputes in the health sector.

The Observatory has made human resources for health a visible policy priority through direct technical cooperation within and among countries.

Source: PAHO 2004b; Rigoli and Arteaga 2004.

user groups. This would involve crafting manuals of key methodologies, policy and operational guidelines, and educational material to accelerate the application of good practices. Technical information on human resource policy and management for categorical programs is already available, as for integrated child health, maternal health, immunization, and treating HIV/AIDS. But very little of such information, either written or digital, is available for human resources in health. These materials should be produced and regularly updated to reflect improving standards of practice under changing circumstances (see the Action & Learning Initiative in chapter 5).

Regional and subregional networks for sharing information on health workforce issues can be found around the world, such as the Commonwealth Regional Health Community Secretariat and the Support for Analysis and Research in Africa project. The internet also enables field workers to communicate with each other—sharing lessons, posing questions, providing answers, and offering professional support in peer dialogue and exchange.[39] For example, the Health Systems Trust, a nongovernmental organization in South Africa, operates a website to support and promote dialogue among health workers dispersed in the country.

Workers in remote locations should be able to connect to such a wealth of information. The findings could be expanded into a evidence-based database on human resources, similar to the Cochrane Database of Systematic Reviews that provides high-quality information to people providing and receiving clinical care.[40] Another example of knowledge sharing, bridging the digital divide, is the Health InterNetwork Access to Research Initiative, which provides health professionals and researchers in low-income countries with free or concessional access to an internet-based library of the latest information on public health.[41]

Strengthening the knowledge base

A stronger knowledge base on human resources requires routine data collection, data harmonization, and research. Health information systems that collect, analyze, report, and use up-to-date health information are necessary for generating, managing, and disseminating knowledge on the health workforce. They provide a platform for decisionmaking by health-care managers, local and national policymakers, and global organizations. The steady building of the knowledge base is a public good that expands the foundation for more effective action.

A solid information system on the workforce is required in all countries. Information on the stock of

> **❝ Far too much of the evidence base for workforce decisionmaking is poor in quality and low in relevance**

workers should include numbers, types, locations, and functions, supplemented by data on level of activity (full-time, part-time), workforce inflow (production, in-migration) and outflow (retirement, death, out-migration). Time trends are particularly helpful for tracking developments. An overhaul of international standards would accelerate national developments by adopting a broad approach to the full spectrum of workers beyond simply counting doctors and nurses. Critical additions are tracking community and other auxiliaries, incorporating a gender lens, and linking worker attributes to health system performance.

Human resource research can build on research groups for health systems. Customarily led and staffed by economists, these groups have developed strong analytical capabilities for tracking the financing of health systems. Policy and management of the workforce should be added to the prevailing economic focus. The challenge should not be underestimated because each resource, human and financial, calls for different assumptions about what makes for better health system performance.

Data gathering and analysis should strive for quality and relevance. Hundreds of workforce studies collect dust on shelves in ministries of health because they lack practicality. Far too much of the evidence base for workforce decisionmaking is poor in quality and low in relevance. Too often, research findings are based on assumptions or anecdotes. Look at the research on short-term training. Many donors and programs focus on short-term training to raise the skill level of workers for performing priority tasks. Recent research suggests that simple training does not generate better practices. Workers rarely practice what they are taught unless

their training is reinforced by supervision and incentives.[42] In other words, training is only one ingredient in changing attitudes and behaviors.

Financing: investing wisely

Like those for workers and knowledge, international financial flows can strengthen—or weaken—a nation's workforce. Development assistance for health, although only a small part of global health spending, is significant in some countries, exceeding half of national health expenditures. How can these flows strengthen national workforces and improve global health equity?

After a decade of decline, foreign aid turned around, swinging up at the turn of the century. By 2002 official development assistance was at $57 billion a year, or 0.23 percent of the gross national income of OECD countries, about a third of the UN-agreed benchmark of 0.7 percent.[43] Health constituted about 13 percent of ODA in 2002, totaling $8.1 billion, significantly higher than $6.4 billion a year in 1997–99 (table 4.1). Bilateral assistance for health increased to $3 billion, with the largest three funders—the United States, Japan, and the United Kingdom—accounting for nearly two-thirds. Funds from UN agencies totaled about $2 billion, about half from the WHO. Development banks channeled another $1.4 billion. The Bill & Melinda Gates Foundation has emerged in the ranks of the largest sources of financing, public or private, for global health.

The human resources share of development assistance for health is unknown, because donors do not classify funding in this category, a reflection of the low priority assigned to the workforce. Strategically, human resource funding should

4

❝ Assuming that development assistance
for health now approaches $10 billion per
year, about $4 billion is for human resources

Table 4.1	Recent trends in development assistance for health (US$ millions)		
		1997–99 average	**2002**
Bilateral agencies		2,559.8	2,875.2
USAID		920.8	1,134.9
Multilateral agencies		3,401.5	4,649.2
UN system		1,575.5	2,036.3
WHO		864.2	1,140.5
Regular budget		406.1	461.1
Extrabudgetary contributions		458.1	776.5
PAHO (own funds)		84.3	93.4
UNAIDS		58.2	91.9
UNICEF		275.8	391.0
UNFPA		293.0	319.5
Development banks		1,522.0	1,405.5
World Bank		1,124.9	983.0
IDA		713.5	536.4
IBRD		411.4	446.6
IADB		245.7	205.0
ADB		287.0	0
AfDB		151.4	217.5
Other multilateral		304.1	1,207.4
European Community		304.1	244.5
Global Fund to Fight AIDS, Tuberculosis, and Malaria		0	962.8
Private nonprofit			
Bill & Melinda Gates Foundation		458.0	595.9
Total development assistance for health		**6,419.3**	**8,120.3**

Source: Michaud 2003.

for health is classified as medical education/ training and health personnel development.[44] But this grossly underestimates large workforce expenditures embedded in program budgets.

Detailed examination of donor reports, program expenditures, and national health accounts by the JLI suggests that a conservative estimate of 40 percent of development assistance for health is for human resources. Assuming that development assistance for health now approaches $10 billion per year, this would translate into about $4 billion for human resources (figure 4.4).[45]

Geographically, the dominant share of this funding goes to sub-Saharan Africa. The share for salaries, training, and technical assistance is more difficult to decipher. Against customary policies, some donors, especially those financing categorical programs, are increasingly funding salaries, allowances, and incentive payments. But the staff of international agencies and technical advisors and consultants command a major share of budgets. Financing for short-term training is also a large part of program budgets, while pre-service educational investments are modest.

Business as usual by donors cannot achieve the MDGs, and efforts to enhance the performance of donor funds will confront three major challenges. The first challenge is policy coherence. In health crisis countries, there is an urgent priority to rapidly scale up life-saving interventions and rebuild crumbling health systems. Donors are proposing large infusions of funds but coordinated policy directions are lacking. The MDGs may have become policy priorities for most donor agencies, but they have yet to encourage greater donor coordination and synergy. And while

include all skill-based human functioning in health systems—for salaries, allowances, and benefits, for education and training, for technical assistance, and for capacity building. Data from the Development Assistance Committee (DAC) of the OECD show that only 1 percent of development assistance

❝❝ Increasing synergies and reducing tensions among categorical priorities are central to strengthening the workforce for achieving national health goals

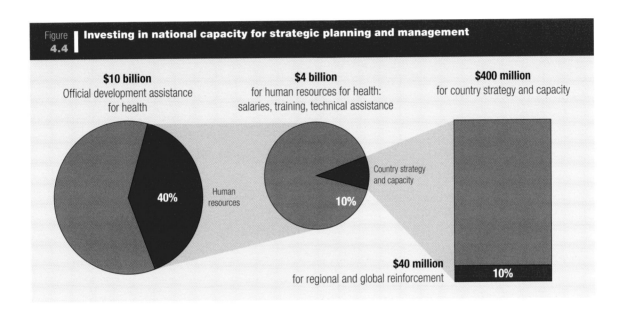

Figure 4.4 | **Investing in national capacity for strategic planning and management**

$10 billion
Official development assistance for health

$4 billion
for human resources for health: salaries, training, technical assistance

$400 million
for country strategy and capacity

40% — Human resources

10% — Country strategy and capacity

$40 million
for regional and global reinforcement

10%

some countries are experiencing explosive growth in funding, other crisis countries are largely overlooked.

A second challenge is harmonizing investments in categorical programs with health system development. Donors are proposing large infusions of HIV/AIDS funding, but systemwide investments have yet to crystallize. Grant funds to address HIV/AIDS were estimated at $5 billion in 2003, and projections suggest that they could increase to $20 billion by 2007.[46] Similarly, the MDGs tend to bias action towards direct programs, not system development. Poorly planned and narrowly executed, categorical programs can destabilize health systems: the deserted health facilities on national immunization days in Madagascar are well documented.[47] Concerns are growing that intensive HIV/AIDS campaigns will produce similar distortions.

Given severe worker shortages, some donors are reportedly offering higher per diem rates to entice workers to join their programs, and others are considering extra incentive pay for their priority

tasks. But giving incentives to only one part of a nation's workforce can undermine motivation and performance of the overall system. That is why increasing synergies and reducing underproductive tensions among disparate priorities in the health sector are central to strengthening workforces and achieving national health goals.[48]

The third challenge is to correct for macroeconomic policies that fail to produce a financial environment for workforce development. Legitimately concerned about fiscal discipline, public sector reforms clamped down on public expenditures in the social sectors—salaries were capped, hiring was frozen, and education and training were neglected. Prolonged application of these policies resulted in severe erosion of the human infrastructure for health, from which many countries are only now emerging (box 4.7).[49] Yet public budgets remain hard pressed with public expenditure ceilings and with employment and wage caps still in place. A

> " **Changing donor mindsets is absolutely essential for workforce development in a rapidly changing health sector**

Under the policy guidance of the International Monetary Fund and the World Bank, the Tanzanian government instituted various policies in 1993 to reduce public expenditures. In health, reducing the number of workers aimed at redressing the skill mix in favor of higher skilled staff. The policies thus called for the retrenchment of thousands of mostly unskilled workers. An employment freeze was enforced for the majority of cadres, partially lifted only in 1998 and finally abolished in 2001.

As the number of health professionals declined, the country's population grew from 27 million to 34 million. The ratio of skilled health personnel to population thus dropped from 109 per 100,000 to 71. Moreover, the disease burden grew disproportionately, with the number of AIDS cases more than doubling. According to the staffing norms developed by the ministry of health, the public sector today faces a shortage of 17,500 skilled health professionals.

Training capacities were cut back to match the reduction in demand. In the early years the system produced more graduates than could be absorbed, but the current output is insufficient to compensate for losses among the workforce. Unless the training capacity is enhanced, the workforce will continue to shrink by approximately 1,000 health professionals a year, even if all future graduates are recruited into service.

The reform measures also lacked mechanisms to redress imbalances in the geographical distribution of health workers. Between 1994 and 2001, the inequality index—the relative deviation of regional staff per population ratios from the national average—climbed from 3.9 to 6.0.

Source: Kurowski and others 2004.

review of eight low-income African countries found that bans on recruitment and staffing had been only partially lifted in half of them.[50] In Rwanda the wage bill is still considered beyond affordability, necessitating new staff cuts in the midst of worker shortages. Without lifting macroeconomic ceilings, workforce expansion, salary improvements, and incentive payments will be impossible, no matter what the volume of funds pledged by donors.

The overall goal of financing strategies is to expand the volume of financial flows and to enhance the health yield of existing resources. To increase the impact of donor funds, the main strategies for the workforce are adopting an investment approach, harmonizing priorities, and generating enabling policies.

Adopting an investment approach

Changing donor mindsets is absolutely essential for workforce development in a rapidly changing health sector. Rather than viewing workers as a fiscal burden—an item of recurrent expenditure in national accounts—an investment approach would set high priorities for financing the workforce, adopt a longer time horizon, and focus on national capacity building. The annual wages paid to health workers, which buy their services for that year but not beyond, are indeed an expenditure. But what is often overlooked is that these expenditures on worker salaries, such as investments in capital or stocks, have returns beyond the year in which the money is spent.

Employing health workers today builds the human stock, work experience, and skill base of the future workforce, thus saving on hiring, turnover,

❝ Coordination by donors and national stakeholders offers opportunities for efficiency gains because transaction costs, overlap, waste, and malfunctioning are reduced for system-wide improvements

Box 4.8	Ghana: Initiatives in human resources for health

Ghana and its development partners have worked collaboratively in five-year programs of work through a sector-wide approach (SWAp). The program focuses on human resources for health as one of 10 priority areas, with emphasis on restructuring numbers, distributions and skill mixes, improving professional development programs, and decentralizing staff management. The policy matrix fixes three output indicators: 80 percent of staff receiving in-service training, 70 percent of core staff continuing to work in Ghana three years after graduation, and better interregional and interdistrict distribution of staff.

In 2001 Ghana qualified for the Heavily Indebted Poor Countries Initiative for debt relief—and formulated its Poverty Reduction Strategy, with health as one element of a large and complex agenda. For health, the strategy calls for bridging equity gaps in access to health services. It provides for redistributing health workers to deprived areas and developing more attractive incentive packages. It also foresees decentralizing the management of human resources to the regions.

Ghana and its development partners are coordinating efforts countrywide through the strategy and support for the sector through the health sector-wide approach. Beyond the usual focus (on the level and structure of public expenditure for health within a medium-term expenditure framework), the three annual Poverty Reduction Strategy Credits expected under the World Bank's country assistance strategy put health worker issues on the agenda for national action by macroeconomic policymakers. Ghana has introduced a salary increase of 15 percent to 35 percent of the base salary for all health workers in 55 deprived districts. Additional funds will be used to attract new health workers to these districts.

Source: Ed Elmendorf; World Bank 2003a, 2003b, 2004a.

training, and transaction costs. This return on worker investments is reaped by public and private health care systems and their clients as well as workers themselves. Moreover, the improved health status gained from more efficient investments in health workers—reductions in maternal mortality associated with greater skilled attendance at birth, for example—benefits not only the individuals directly affected but also the social and economic well-being of their families and communities.

An investment approach would harmonize workforce development with other inputs. It would also build a solid foundation for workforce development through development assistance for health that is steady and predictable, rather than episodic or fluctuating. Debt relief under HIPC is

a good mechanism for predictability and stability. Another would be the new International Finance Facility, proposed by the United Kingdom, to have donor commitments through 2015 used as collateral for bonds issued in international capital markets—to provide grants to resource-poor countries.[51] This could be tested and assessed in a small set of countries and scaled up if found effective.

An investment approach would also balance allocations in support of building national capacity— pre-service education not just short-term training, institution building not just technical assistance, national ownership and decisionmaking not just donor-driven activities. Every donor-supported health program should be pursued with an investment plan for human resources, supplemented by a human resource audit.

❝ For the double crisis countries—those facing rising mortality rates with feeble health systems—health donors are entering uncharted waters

Harmonizing priorities

Coordination by donors and national stakeholders offers opportunities for efficiency gains because transaction costs, overlap, waste, and malfunctioning are reduced for system-wide improvements (box 4.8). In addition to procedural coordination, strengthening the workforce itself can be a focal point for coordinating diverse donor activities. Because the workforce is central to all health activities, its development can be a crossroads for donor synchronization—a common currency for the harmonization of disparate donor activities. Coherent workforce development would be a goal as well as a sign of effective donor coordination.

Putting the workforce first may help resolve impending tensions between categorical priority programs and health systems development. Each has a legitimate rationale. Categorical programs have clear missions and targets and invariably require a workforce to produce results. Health systems development builds the human and physical infrastructure for all health activities. To grow and develop in a balanced manner, however, health systems require the cooperation and investment of all programs, including the categorical. Earmarked financing to achieve specific outputs within an overall health systems framework promotes accountability and reduces resource diversions and leakages.

Opportunities for synergy between the two must be seized at the country level. A win-win approach recognizes that the sustainability of categorical programs ultimately depends on the strength of the overall health system. Moreover, the broader range of services offered by health systems may enhance the effectiveness of categorical programs. The treatment coverage of HIV-positive Haitians has reportedly been accelerated as eligible candidates are attracted to a range of basic services provided in primary health care facilities.[52] In parallel, health system performance can be improved with clearer policies for key problems and the specification of time-bound outputs. Setting discrete targets for priority problems helps align and energize health systems to deliver results under constrained circumstances.

Ultimately, harmonization between categorical programs and health systems is a political-technical process in diverse countries. How much of these systems should be narrowly focused to priority diseases? What are the policies, practices, and investment priorities of host countries? National ownership of the investment strategy, appropriate funding matched to local needs, and the commitment and capacity of national stakeholders should guide the harmonization.[53]

Generating enabling policies

Workforce development depends on public budgets to create posts, pay salaries, and finance incentive payments (chapter 3). Achieving national health goals, such as the MDGs, will require a doubling or tripling of workers in many of the poorest countries.[54] Macroeconomic policies are thus essential for workforce development. For the double crisis countries—those facing rising mortality rates with feeble health systems—health donors are entering uncharted waters. Creativity and innovation will be required to manage the vastly greater resources needed. Macroeconomic policies must expand the resource envelope, massively in some cases, and the workforce must grow in sync with drugs, supplies, and transport. Sheer numeric deficiencies must be overcome through mobilization and training for scaling up activities.

> **Macroeconomic frameworks must be adjusted to allow countries to make greater and longer term investments in the health workforce**

Box 4.9 | **Worker-friendly donor policies**

Traditional policies

Funding
- A recurrent expenditure
- Earmarked, restricted
- Fragmentation of funds
- Procedurally oriented

Time horizon
- Brief, repeated commitments
- Short-term training

Operations
- Focus on drugs, financing
- Priority disease control
- Foreign technical assistance
- Little monitoring and evaluation

Worker-friendly policies

Funding
- A leveraging investment
- Flexible, fungible
- Coordination, pooling of funds
- Outcome and capacity-oriented

Time horizon
- Sustained investment horizons
- Educational institution capacity and continuous learning

Operations
- Focus on worker retention
- Health systems performance
- National capacity building
- HRH monitoring/impact assessment

Major infusions of donor funds will be necessary to tackle the double crisis. Yet many recipient countries may lack the absorptive capacity to apply these funds. Already, field reports suggest a growing backlog of donor expenditures in relation to commitments—which some attribute to weak national capacity to use external funds. Cited is the lack of efficient administrative and financial procedures to disburse donor funds. While the concerns have some validity, the obstacles surely differ in diverse countries.

In some countries, absorption problems exhibit some Catch-22 dilemmas. Chronic underinvestment in human resources means that fewer skilled people are able to use donor funds expeditiously, a vicious cycle. Such underinvestments, which only deplete national capacity, should not be allowed to shift blame for current difficulties. Indeed, greater sustained investment in human resources can overcome absorption constraints.

Absorption problems are also due to misfits between internal and external factors. Donor procedures and conditions are still far from optimal for internal implementation. Weak absorption may be a consequence of inappropriate investments—for example, targeting donor funds to low priority or impractical activities. Donors often assume the availability of complementary inputs for their projects, such as staff or time or systems, which together over-tax and overwhelm national systems. Practical solutions to absorptive capacity should be developed with creativity and flexibility on a country-by-country basis.

Macroeconomic frameworks must be adjusted to allow countries to make greater and longer term investments in the health workforce. The challenge is to create "workforce-friendly" macroeconomic policies (chapter 3 and box 4.9).

> **❝ The ultimate responsibility of actors at the global level is to undertake the range of reinforcing actions that contribute to the success of national strategies**

Conclusion

Flows of workers, knowledge, and finance have positive and negative potentialities for the health workforce. The policy challenge is to mitigate the harm while harnessing the benefits.

Who has the responsibility for managing these flows? Each is distinctive, each with its own community of actors. Medical migration is of interest to national governments, professional councils and societies, nongovernmental organizations, and workers and their families. Knowledge producers, users, and brokers are in academia, universities, educational institutions, and various technical agencies. Ensuring the collection and dissemination of key information will generate public awareness and political commitment from leaders to strengthen the health workforce and enhance health and accountability. Concessional international financing is governed and managed by donor and recipient governments, multilateral organizations, and civil society groups.

Responsibility thus must be shared among these actor groups, extending beyond national health sectors alone. The impact on the health workforce of global actors in health financing and trade can be as strong as that of local institutions—and as such, actors must be engaged in workforce development at all levels, national, regional, global. Particularly promising opportunities for collaboration and exchange can be developed at the regional level. In the realm of education, for example, regional bodies such as CAMES in Francophone Africa (the African and Madagascan Council for Higher Education) and PAHO in the Americas (the Pan-American Health Organization) have created and managed regionally relevant training initiatives, exchange programs, and accreditation schemes. Neighborly exchange of workers with similar cultural and linguistic traditions could also help equilibrate imbalances. And opportunities for shared and joint financing of other workforce developments—such as data collection or knowledge management—could also be explored.

Global institutions, no matter how successful, have little effect without local capacity. Ultimately, it is capacity at local, national and regional levels together that determines the effective translation of global developments. The ultimate responsibility of actors at the global level is to undertake the range of reinforcing actions that contribute to the success of national strategies.

Notes

1. Ncayiyana 1999.
2. African Union 2003.
3. Biviano and Makarehchi 2002.
4. Dovlo 2003.
5. Buerhaus and others 2000.
6. Mareckova 2004.
7. Buchan and others 2003.
8. BBC 2003b.
9. Dugger 2004.
10. Franco and others 2002; Peters and others 2002; Franco and others 2004.
11. PAHO 2001; Xaba and Phillips 2001; Lorenzo 2002.
12. Mutume 2003.
13. Dovlo and Martineau 2004.
14. Dovlo and Nyonator 1999.
15. Rigoli and Dussault 2003.
16. Kurowski and others 2003.
17. Health Canada 2004.
18. O'Hagan 2002; Thompson 2001.
19. Buerhaus and others 2000; Department of Health 2002; O'Hagan 2002.
20. Buchan and Dovlo 2004.
21. OECD 2004.
22. Heller and Mills 2002; Dovlo and Martineau 2004.
23. Jayaram 1995.
24. OECD 2003.
25. Daar 2004.
26. Ratha 2003.
27. Lucas 2001.

28. Gaillard and Gaillard 1998; Meyer and Brown 1999; Turner and others 2003.
29. Curran and others 2004.
30. Wibulpolprasert and others 2004.
31. UNCTAD and WHO 1998.
32. Chaudhuri and others 2004.
33. Deaton 2004.
34. WHO 2000.
35. Pablos-Mendez and Brown 2004.
36. Berwick 2003.
37. Barnett and Whiteside 2002.
38. Health Metrics Network 2004.
39. Health Metrics Network 2004.
40. Update Software 2004.
41. Health InterNetwork 2004.
42. Grol and Grimshaw 2003; Das and Hammer 2004.
43. Michaud 2003.
44. Goel 2003.
45. This estimation was done for JLI by Catherine Michaud in 2004 based on the OECD/CRS online database available at [www.oecd.org/dac/stats/crs/].
46. UNAIDS 2004.
47. Oliveira-Cruz and others 2003.
48. Council on Foreign Relations and Milbank Memorial Fund 2004.
49. Liese and Dussault 2004.
50. Kurowski and others 2004.
51. Gehmlich 2004.
52. Walton and others 2004.
53. Glenngard and Anell 2003.
54. Kurowski 2004a.

References

African Development Bank. 2002. *Achieving the Millennium Development Goals in Africa: Progress, Prospects and Policy Implications*. Abidjan.

African Union. 2003. Conference of the African Ministers of Health, "Investing in Health for Africa's Socioeconomic Development," Seventh Session, April 26–30, Tripoli.

Barnett, T., and A. Whiteside. 2002. *AIDS in the 21st Century: Disease and Globalization*. London: Macmillan.

BBC News. 2002. "NHS Poaching Third World Nurses." November 26.

———. 2003a. "NHS Still Relies on Overseas Nurses." May 12.

———. 2003b. "Nurses Exodus." August 27.

Berwick, D. 2002. "A Learning World for the Global Fund." *British Medical Journal* 325 (7355): 55–56.

———. 2003. "Disseminating Innovations in Health Care." *Journal of the American Medical Association* 289 (15): 1969–75.

Biviano, M., and F. Makarehchi. 2002. "Globalization and the Physician Workforce in the United States." Presented at the Sixth International Medical Workforce Conference, April 25, Ottawa.

Bourne, Peter G., and Gail Reed. 2003a. Interview with Dr. Jaime Davis, head of the Cuban medical team in South Africa, July 17, Johannesburg.

———. 2003b. Interview with Dr. Yiliam Jiménez, Director, Comprehensive Health Program. October 17, Havana.

Buchan, J. 2002. "International Recruitment of Nurses: United Kingdom Case Study." Royal College of Nursing, London. [Retrived on October 8, 2004, from www.rcn.org.uk/publications/pdf/irn-case-study-booklet.pdf].

Buchan, J., and D. Dovlo. 2004. "International Recruitment of Health Workers to the UK: A Report to DFID." DFID Health Systems Resource Centre, London.

Buchan, James, Tina Parkin, and Julie Sochalski. 2003. "International Nurse Mobility. Trends and Policy Implications." World Health Organization, International Council of Nurses, Royal College of Nursing, Geneva.

Buerhaus, P., D. Staiger, and D. Auerbach. 2000. "Implications of Rapidly Aging Nurse Workforce." *Journal of the American Medical Association* 283 (22): 2948–54.

Castles, S. 2000. "International Migration at the Beginning of the Twenty-First Century: Global Trends and Issues." *International Migration* 52 (165): 269–83.

Castro, F. 2003. Speech at national medical school graduation ceremonies, August 13, Havana. Unpublished transcript.

Chan, Danny. 2003. "Philippine Doctors Study Nursing to Land U.S. Jobs." SikhSpectrum.com Issue 10. [Retrieved October 8, 2004, from www.sikhspectrum.com/].

Chaudhuri, Sumanta, Aaditya Mattoo, and Richard Self. 2004. "Moving People to Deliver Services: How Can the WTO Help?" Policy Research Working Paper 3238. World Bank, Washington, D.C.

Commonwealth Secretariat. 2002. "Commonwealth Code of Practice for International Recruitment of Health Workers." Draft. London.

Council on Foreign Relations and Milbank Memorial Fund. 2004. *Addressing the HIV/AIDS Pandemic: A U.S. Global AIDS Strategy for the Long-Term*. Milbank Memorial Fund. New York.

Curran, James, Haile Debas, Monisha Arya, Patrick Kelley, Stacey Knobler, and Leslie Pray, eds. 2004. *Scaling Up Treatment for the Global AIDS Pandemic: Challenges and Opportunities*. Washington, D.C.: National Academy of Sciences.

Daar, Abdallah. 2004. "Diaspora Options: How

Developing Countries Could Benefit from Their Emigrant Populations." University of Toronto, Joint Center for Bioethics, Canada.

Das, J., and J. Hammer. 2004. "Strained Mercy: The Quality of Medical Care in Delhi." Policy Research Working Paper 3228. World Bank, Washington, D.C.

Davila, Carlos Lage. 2001. Speech of the Cuban Vice President at UN Meeting on AIDS, June 25, New York.

Deaton, Angus. 2004. "Health in an Age of Globalization." Draft. Prepared for the Brooking Trade Forum, Brookings Institution, May 13–14, Washington, D.C.

Department of Health, United Kingdom. 2001. *Code of Practice for NHS Employers Involved in International Recruitment of Health Care Professionals*. London.

———. 2002. *Delivering the NHS Plan: Next Steps on Investment, Next Steps on Reform*. London.

Department for International Development. 2003. "Promoting Institutional and Organisational Development: A Sourcebook of Tools and Techniques." London. [Retrieved October 8, 2004, from www.dfid.gov.uk/pubs/files/prominstdevsourcebook.pdf].

Dewdney, J. 2001. *The WPRO/RTC Health Workforce Planning Workbook*. Centre for Public Health, The University of New South Wales, Sydney. [Retrieved October 8, 2004, from http://hrhtoolkit.forumone.com/planania/mstr_planania_workbook.pdf].

Dovlo, D. 1999. "Report on Issues Affecting the Mobility and Retention of Health Workers in Commonwealth African States." Commonwealth Secretariat, Arusha, Tanzania.

———. 2003. Background Paper for Consultative Workshop on Human Resources for Health in East Central and Southern Africa, July 21–25, Arusha, Tanzania.

Dovlo, Delanyo, and Tim Martineau. 2004. "Review of Evidence for Push and Pull Factors and Impact on Health Worker Mobility in Africa." Joint Learning Initiative Working Paper. Ghana and Liverpool School of Tropical Medicine, United Kingdom. [www.globalhealthtrust.org/].

Dovlo, D., and F. Nyator. 1999. "Migration of Graduates of the University of Ghana Medical School: A Preliminary Rapid Appraisal." *Human Resources for Health Development Journal* 3 (1): 34–37.

Dugger, Celia W. 2004. "An Exodus of African Nurses Puts Infants and the Ill in Peril." *New York Times*, July 12.

Dumont, J. C., and J. B. Meyer. 2004. "The International Mobility of Health Professionals: An Evaluation and Analysis Based on the Case of South Africa." Part III. From *Trends in International Migration: SOPEMI 2003*. Paris: Organisation for Economic Co-operation and Development.

Dussault, G., and M. Franceschini. 2003. "Not Enough Here, Too Many There: Understanding Geographical Imbalances in the Distribution of the Health Workforce." World Bank, Washington, D.C.

Editorial. 2000. "Medical Migration and Inequity of Health Care." *The Lancet* 356 (9225): 177.

Egger, D., D. Lipson, and O. Adams. 2000. "Achieving the Right Balance: The Role of Policy-Making Processes in Managing Human Resources for Health Problems. " Issues in Health Services Delivery. Human Resources for Health. Discussion Paper 2. World Health Organisation, Geneva.

Franco, L., S. Bennett, and R. Kanfer. 2002. "Health Sector Reform and Public Sector Health Worker Motivation: A Conceptual Framework." *Social Science and Medicine* 54 (8): 1255–66.

Franco, L., S. Bennett, R. Kanfer, and P. Stubblebine. 2004. "Determinants and Consequences of Health Worker Motivation in Hospitals in Jordan and Georgia." *Social Science and Medicine* 58 (2): 343–55.

Fülöp, T., and M. Roemer. 1987. *Reviewing Health Manpower Development: A Method of Improving National Health Systems*. World Health Organization, Geneva.

Gaillard, J., and A. Gaillard. 1998. "The International Circulation of Scientists and Technologists: A Win-Lose or Win-Win Situation." *Science Communication* 20 (1): 106–115.

Gehmlich, K. 2004. "Paris, London Urge Deal to Double Third World Aid." Reuters News.

Glenngård, Anna, and Anders Anell. 2003. "Investment in Human Resources for Health—Problems, Approaches and Donor Experiences." Joint Learning Initiative Working Paper. The Swedish Institute for Health Economics. [www.globalhealthtrust.org/].

Goel, Shashank. 2003. "Memo on Investments Flows in HRH." Global Equity Initiative, Harvard University, Cambridge, Mass.

Grol, R., and J. Grimshaw. 2003. "From Best Evidence to Best Practice: Effective Implementation of Change in Patient's Care." *The Lancet* 362 (9391): 1225–30.

Hagopian, Amy, Anthony Ofosu, Adesegun Fatusi, Richard Biritwum, Ama Essel, L. Gary Hart, and Carolyn Watts. "The Flight of Physicians from West Africa: Views of African Physicians and Implications for Policy." Draft. Submitted for publication to *Social Science and Medicine*.

Haines, Andy, and Andrew Cassels. 2004. "Can the Millennium Development Goals Be Attained?" *British Medical Journal* 329 (7462): 394–97.

Hall, T. 2001a. "Guidelines for a HRH Review." World Health Organization, Geneva. [Retrieved October

8, 2004, from http://hrhtoolkit.forumone.com].

———. 2001b. "Simulation Models for Workforce Planning." World Health Organization, Geneva. [Retrieved October 8, 2004, from http://hrhtoolkit.forumone.com].

Hall, T. L., and A. Goubarev. 2000. "Information Technology and Human Resources Development: The World Health Organization's HRD ToolKit." *Human Resources Development Journal* 4(1). [Retrieved October 8, 2004, from www.moph.go.th/ops/hrdj/hrdj9/pdf9/Tom41.pdf].

Health Canada. 2004. "Health Human Resources: Balancing Supply and Demand." *Health Policy Research Bulletin* 8. [Retrieved October 8, 2004, from www.hc-sc.gc.ca/iacb-dgiac/arad-draa/english/rmdd/bulletin/ehuman.pdf].

Health InterNetwork. 2004. *HINARI.* [Retrieved October 8, 2004, from www.healthinternetwork.org/].

Health Metrics Network. 2004. "Working Together to Improve Health Information for Health Action." Executive Summary and Business Plan. Unpublished document prepared during the development phase of the Health Metrics Network. World Health Organization, Geneva.

Heller, P. S., and A. Mills. 2002. "The Brain Drain—Health Workers Here and There." *International Herald Tribune*, July 25.

ILO (International Labour Organization). 2000. *Migration: A Truly Global Phenomenon.* Geneva.

Jayaram, N. 1995. "The Political Economy of Medical Education in India." *Higher Education Policy* 8 (2): 29–32.

Kurowski, Christoph. 2004a. "Scope, Characteristics and Policy Implications of the Health Worker Shortage in Low-Income Countries of Sub-Saharan Africa." Joint Learning Initiative Working Paper. World Bank, Washington, D.C. [www.globalhealthtrust.org/].

———. 2004b. "Increasing the Effectiveness of Spending on Human Resources for Health: A Proposal for Strategic Planning." Working Paper. World Bank, Washington, D.C.

Kurowski, Christoph, Sonia Ruiz, Anna Dominick, and Anne Mills. 2004. "A Decade of Fiscal Stabilization in Tanzania—Its Impact on the Performance of the Health Workforce." Working Paper. London School of Hygiene and Tropical Medicine, London.

Kurowski, Christoph, Kaspar Wyss, Salim Abdulla, N'Diekhor Yémadji, and Anne Mills. 2003. "Human Resources for Health: Requirements and Availability in the Context of Scaling Up Priority Interventions in Low-Income Countries. Case Studies from Tanzania and Chad." Working Paper. London School of Hygiene and Tropical Medicine, London.

Liese, Bernhard, and Gilles Dussault. 2004. "The Human Resource Crisis in Health Services in Sub-Saharan Africa." World Bank, Washington, D.C.

Lorenzo, F. 2002. "Nurse Supply and Demand in the Philippines." Institute of Health Policy and Development Studies, University of the Philippines, Manila.

Lowell, B. L. 2001. *Policy Responses to the International Mobility of Skilled Labour.* International Migration Papers 45. International Labour Office, International Migration Branch. Geneva. [www.ilo.org/public/english/protection/migrant/download/imp/imp45.pdf].

———. 2002. *Some Development Effects of the International Migration of Highly Skilled Persons.* International Migration Papers 46. International Labour Office, International Migration Branch. Geneva. [Retrieved October 14, 2004, from www.ilo.org/public/english/protection/migrant/download/imp/imp46.pdf].

Lowell, B. L., and A. Findlay. 2001. *Migration of Highly Skilled Persons from Developing Countries: Impact and Policy Responses: Synthesis Report.* International Migration Papers 44. International Labour Office, International Migration Branch. Geneva. [Retrieved October 14, 2004, from www.ilo.org/public/english/protection/migrant/download/imp/imp44.pdf].

Lucas, R. 2001. "Diaspora and Development: Highly Skilled Migrants from East Asia. A Report to the World Bank." World Bank, Washington, D.C.

Maamar, Ahmed. 2003. Speech of the Algerian Ambassador to Cuba, May 24, Astral Theater, Havana.

Management Sciences for Health. 2000. "Decentralization Mapping Tool." [Retrieved October 8, 2004, from http://erc.msh.org/mainpage.cfm?file=6.10.htm&module=toolkit&language=English].

———. 2003. "Human Capacity Development (HCD): An Inquiry Based on the HCD Framework developed by the Office of HIV/AIDS, USAID." [http://erc.msh.org/].

Mareckova, Martina. 2004. "Exodus of Czech Doctors Leaves Gaps in Health Care." *The Lancet* 363 (9419): 1443–46.

Martineau, T., and J. Martinez. 1997. *Human Resources in the Health Sector: Guidelines for Appraisal and Strategic Development.* European Commission. Brussels. [Retrieved October 8, 2004, from www.liv.ac.uk/lstm/hsr/hrdcover.html].

Martineau, T., K. Decker, and P. Bundred. 2002. "Briefing Note on International Migration of Health Professionals: Leveling the Playing Field for Developing Country Health Systems." Liverpool School of Tropical Medicine, Liverpool, United Kingdom.

Martinez, J., and T. Martineau. 1996. "Human Resources and Health Sector Reforms: Research and Development Priorities in Developing Countries." Workshop on human resources and health sector reforms, "Research and Development Priorities in Developing Countries," August, Liverpool, United Kingdom. International Health Division, LSTM.

———. 1998. "Rethinking Human Resources: An Agenda for the Millennium." *Health Policy and Planning* 13 (4): 345–58.

Meyer, J., and M. Brown. 1999. "Scientific Diasporas: A New Approach to Brain Drain." United Nations Educational, Scientific and Cultural Organization, Paris.

Michaud, Catherine. 2003. "Development Assistance for Health: Recent Trends and Resource Allocation." World Health Organization, Geneva.

Ministry of Foreign Relations, Cuba. Undated. *Globalizando la solidaridad.* Programa Integral de Salud.

———. 2004. "Comprehensive Health Program Database." Departamento de Cooperación Internacional, Havana.

Ministry of Foreign Relations and the Vice Ministry for Medical Education, Cuba. 2004. Data from the Comprehensive Health Program and International Cooperation Office. Office of Foreign Student Enrollment, Havana.

Ministry of Public Health, Cuba. 2003a. "Datos Históricos de la Cooperación Médica." Unidad de Colaboración Médica, Havana.

———. 2003b. Country reports from Cuban medical teams. Unidad de Colaboración Médica, Havana.

———. 2003c. Unidad de Colaboración Médica database. Unidad de Colaboración Médica, Havana.

———. 2004a. "Datos Históricos de la Cooperación Médica." Unidad de Colaboración Médica, Havana.

———. 2004b. "Tablas de Colaboracion, 2003." Memo from Dr. R. Bagarotti. Unidad de Colaboración Médica, Havana.

Ministry of Health, Ghana. 2003. *Human Resource Strategy.* Accra.

Moore, M. 2003. "What Does Globalization Mean?" In *A World Without Walls. Freedom, Development, Free Trade and Global Governance.* Cambridge: Cambridge University Press.

Mutume, G. 2003. "Reversing Africa's Brain Drain." *Africa Recovery* 17 (2): 1–9.

National Library of Medicine. 2004. PubMed. Bethesda, Md. [Retrieved October 8, 2004, from www.ncbi.nlm.nih.gov/entrez/query.fcgi].

Ncayiyana, D. 1999. "Doctor Migration is a Universal Phenomenon." *South African Medical Journal* 89 (11): 1107.

OECD (Organisation for Economic Co-operation and Development). 2004. "Database on Aid Activities." [www.oecd.org/dac/stats/crs/].

———. 2000. *Trends in International Migration.* Paris.

———. 2002. "International Migration of Physicians and Nurses: Causes, Consequences and Health Policy Implications." Draft. Paris.

———. 2003. "The DAC Journal Development Co-operation Report 2002—Efforts and Policies of the Members of the Development Assistance Committee." *The DAC Journal* 4 (1): I–323.

———. 2004. "The International Mobility of Health Professionals: An Evaluation and Analysis Based on the Case of South Africa." In *Trends in International Migration, SOPEMI 2003 Edition.* Paris.

O'Hagan, J. 2002. "Turning the Tide." *Sydney Morning Herald,* October 2.

Oliveira-Cruz, O., C. Kurowski, and A. Mills. 2003. "Delivery of Priority Health Services: Searching for Synergies within the Vertical versus Horizontal Debate." *Journal of International Development* 15 (1): 67–86.

O'Neill, M. 2001. Human Resource Development (HRD) Assessment Instrument for NGOs and Public Sector Health Organizations, Management Sciences for Health. [Retrieved October 8, 2004, from http://erc.msh.org/].

Pablos-Mendez, Ariel, and Hilary Brown. 2004. "Knowledge Management in Public Health." Joint Learning Initiative Working Paper. World Health Organization, Geneva, and the Rockefeller Foundation, New York. [Retrieved October 8, 2004, from www.globalhealthtrust.org/doc/abstracts/WG6/MendezBrownFINAL.pdf].

Padarath, Ashnie, Charlotte Chamberlain, David McCoy, Antoinette Ntuli, Mike Rowson, and Rene Loewenson. 2003. "Health Personnel in Southern Africa: Confronting Maldistribution and Brain Drain." Equinet Disscussion Paper 3. Harare.

PAHO (Pan American Health Organization). 2001. "Report on the Technical Meeting on Managed Migration of Skilled Nursing Personnel." Caribbean Office, Bridgetown, Barbados.

———. 2004a. "Observatory of Human Resources." [Retrieved October 8, 2004, at www.lachsr.org/observatorio/eng/index.html].

———. 2004b. "Observatory of Human Resources in Health, 134th Session of the Executive Committee." June 21–25. Washington, D.C. [Retrieved October 8, 2004, from www.paho.org/common/Display.asp?Lang=E&RecID=6620].

Peters, David H., Abdo S. Yazbeck, Rashmi R. Sharma, G. N. V. Ramana, Lant H. Pritchett, and Adam Wagstaff. 2002. "Better Health Systems for India's Poor: Findings, Analysis and Options." World Bank, Washington, D.C.

Rai, S. 2003. "Indian Nurses Sought to Staff U.S. Hospitals: Exams Cover Medicine and U.S. Culture." New York Times, February 10.

Ratha, D. 2003. "Worker's Remittances: An Important and Stable Source of External Development Finance." *Global Development Finance: Striving for Stability in Development Finance*. Vol. 1. Washington, D.C.: World Bank.

Reed, G. A. 2000. "Challenges for Cuba's Family Doctor-and-Nurse Program." *MEDICC Review* 11(3).

Rigoli, Félix, and Oscar Arteaga. 2004. "The Experience of the Latin America and Caribbean Observatory of Human Resources in Health." Joint Learning Initiative Working Paper. Pan American Health Organization, El Paso, Tex., Universidad de Chile, Santiago. [www.globalhealthtrust.org/].

Rigoli, Felix, and Gilles Dussault. 2003. "The Interface between Health Sector Reform and Human Resources for Health." *Human Resources for Health* 1(9).

San Francisco Chronicle. 2003. "Doctors Leaving Philippines to Become Nurses—For the Money." November 5.

Sepulveda, J., ed. 2002. *Panamerican Health in the 21st Century—Strengthening International Cooperation and Development of Human Capital*. Cuernavaca, Mexico: National Institute of Public Health.

Stalker, P. 2000. *Workers Without Frontiers: The Impact of Globalization on International Migration*. Geneva: Lynne Rienner Publishers.

Thompson, Pamela. 2001. "Wanted: U.S. 'Reinvestment' to Help Recruit, Retrain Nurses." *AHA News*, July 30, 2001. American Hospitals Association, Chicago. [Retrieved October 8, 2004, from www.aha.org/ahanews/jsp/ahanews.jsp?Action=30-Jul-2001].

Turner, William, Claude Henry, and Mamadou Gueye. 2003. "Diasporas, Development and Information and Communication Technologies." In R. Barre, V. Hernandez, J. Meyer, and D. Vinck., eds., *Diasporas scientifiques. Expertise collegiales: Institute de Recherche sur le Developpement*. Ministere des Affaires Etrangeres. Paris.

UNAIDS (Joint United Nations Programme on HIV/AIDS). 2004. *2004 Report on the Global AIDS Epidemic: 4th Global Report*. Geneva.

UNCTAD (United Nations Conference on Trade and Development) and WHO (World Health Organization). 1998. "International Trade in Health Services. A Development Perspective." Geneva.

UNDP (United Nations Development Programme). 2003a. *Human Development Report 2003: Millennium Development Goals: A Compact Among Nations to End Human Poverty*. New York: Oxford University Press.

———. 2003b. *Informe Sobre Desarrollo Humano, 2003*. Mundi-Prensa. [http://hdr.undp.org/reports/].

Update Software. 2004. *Cochrane Library*. [Retrieved October 8, 2004, from www.update-software.com/cochrane/].

Vujicic, M., P. Zurn, K. Diallo, O. Adams, and M. R. Dal Poz. 2004. "The Role of Wages in the Migration of Health Care Professionals from Developing Countries." *Human Resources for Health* 2(3).

Wagstaff, Adam, and Marium Claeson. 2004. *The Millennium Development Goals for Health—Rising to the Challenges*. World Bank. Washington, D.C.

Walton, David A., Paul E. Farmer, Wesler Lambert, F. Léandre, Serena P. Koenig, and Joia S. Mukherjee. 2004. "Integrated HIV Prevention and Care Strengthens Primary Health Care: Lessons from Rural Haiti." *Journal of Public Health Policy* 25 (2): 137–58.

Washington Post Foreign Service. 2004. "Filipinos Take 'Going Places' Literally." May 26.

Wenger, E. 1998. *Communities of Practice. Learning, Meaning and Identity*. New York: Cambridge University Press.

WHO (World Health Organization). Undated. "Human Capacity Building for 3 by 5: Country Fact, Planning & Monitoring Sheet." Unpublished document. Geneva.

———. 2000. *World Health Report 2000: Health Systems: Improving Performance*. Geneva.

———. 2003. *International Nurse Mobility—Trends and Policy Implications*. Geneva.

———. 2004. "About Health Metrics Network." [Retrieved October 8, 2004, from www.who.int/healthmetrics/about/en/].

Wibulpolprasert, Suwit, Cha-aim Pachanee, Siriwan Pitayarangsarit, and Pintusorn Hempisut. 2004. "International Service Trade and Its Implication on Human Resources for Health: A Case Study of Thailand." *Human Resources for Health* 2(10).

Willetts, A., and T. Martineau. 2004. *Ethical International Recruitment of Health Professionals: Will Codes of Practice Protect Developing Country Health Systems?* Liverpool School of Tropical Medicine, Liverpool. [Retrieved October 8, 2004, from www.liv.ac.uk/lstm/research/documents/codesofpracticereport.pdf].

World Bank. 1993. *World Development Report 1993: Investing in Health*. New York: Oxford University Press.

———. 2003a. "Ghana Poverty Reduction Strategy—An Agenda for Growth and Prosperity, 2003–2005." Vol. 1. [Retrieved October 6, 2004, from http://siteresources.worldbank.org/GHANAEXTN/Resources/Ghana_PRSP.pdf].

———. 2003b. "Project Appraisal Document on a Proposed Development Credit and Development Grant for a Health Sector Program Support Project II." Human Development II, Africa Regional Office, Report 24842-GH. Washington, D.C.

———. 2004. *Program Document for a Proposed Credit and Grant to Ghana for a Second Poverty*

Reduction Support Credit. Poverty Reduction and Management 4, Africa Region, Report 29177-GH.

Xaba, J., and G. Phillips. 2001. "Understanding Nurse Migration: Final Report." Trade Union Research Project, Pretoria.

Putting workers first

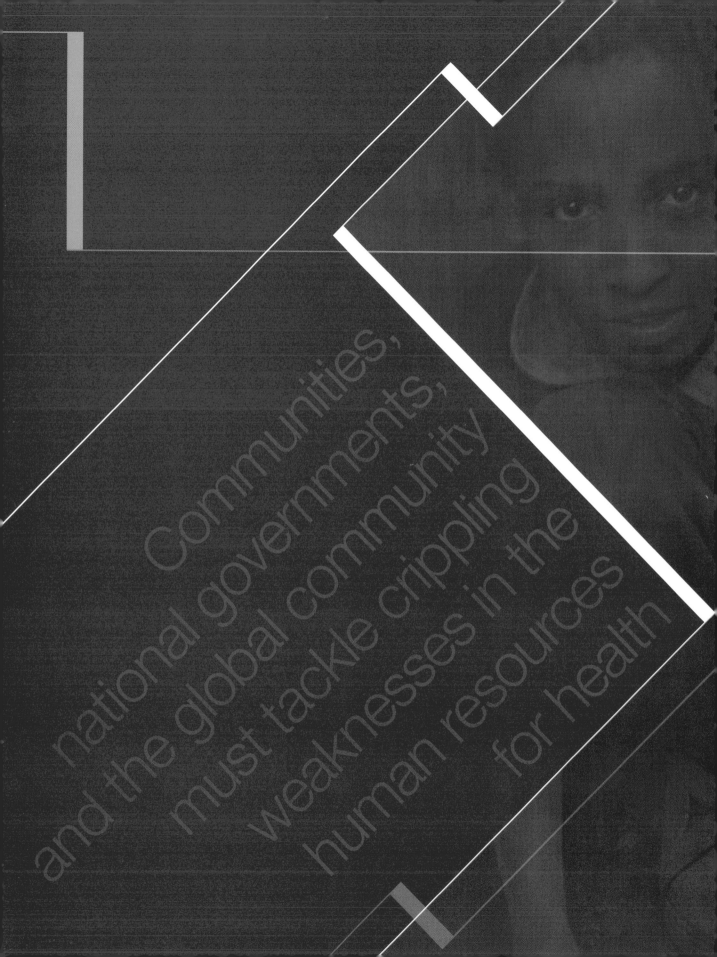

Communities, national governments, and the global community must tackle crippling weaknesses in the human resources for health

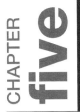

CHAPTER **five**

Putting Workers First

This report offers compelling evidence for action by communities, national governments, and the global community to tackle crippling weaknesses in human resources for health. Overcoming workforce obstacles opens opportunities to strengthen the capacity of health systems to complete the "unfinished health agenda" of the last century, to achieve the health-related Millennium Development Goals (MDGs), and to meet the urgent challenges of HIV/AIDS and other major diseases threatening those at greatest risk.

The imperative for action springs from the urgency of health crises, the timeliness of fresh opportunities, and the prospect that available knowledge, if applied vigorously, could save many lives. The cost of inaction is unmistakable—stark failures to achieve the MDGs, epidemics spiraling out of control, and unnecessary losses of many lives. At stake: nothing less than the course of global health and development in the 21st century.

Exceptional action is indicated for all stakeholder groups. "Business as usual" will simply not do. Although human resources are not a panacea, no successful health action can succeed without an effective workforce. The response at its core must be country-based and country-led—because all global initiatives must be implemented, planned, and owned in specific national settings. The response must be multidimensional. Technical approaches alone will not do, because adequate financing, strong leadership, and political commitment are all necessary. The response must be inclusive, engaging all relevant stakeholders, including non-health and nongovernmental groups. And in the poorest countries, the response must also include appropriate behavior by the international community, because external resources must supplement domestic resources.

> **Every country, poor or rich, should have a national workforce plan to build sustainable health systems for addressing national health needs**

The credibility of existing national, regional, and global health institutions is under siege. Health emergencies, collapsing health systems, and crises in human resources cannot be sealed off to only the poorest countries. These ultimately are global problems. Strengthening the health workforce is a shared challenge that demands commonly developed solutions—a mutual responsibility of all. The key to unlocking our shared health future is to galvanize action by all actors for strengthening human resources in health—to combat health crises and to build sustainable health systems.

Richer countries must aim to achieve self-sufficiency in workforce production to dampen recruitment pressures of health professionals, particularly doctors and nurses from countries already facing worker shortages. Poorer countries must develop strategies to retain their skilled workforces by creating more positive work environments in which workers feel recognized, rewarded, and productive. In many countries, a more appropriate skill mix should be developed, involving cadres of auxiliary community workers. Global programs that seek to tackle priority diseases must integrate workforce development into national priorities. Global institutions, donors, and health policy leaders must elevate the critical importance of human resources for health and develop more coherent policies and technical support for country strategies.

Actions must be pursued over a "decade for human resources for health" (2006–2015) and implemented through alliances for action. Crafting a workforce to meet national health needs requires sustained efforts over time; it cannot be a fleeting fad. This timeline also matches the remaining 10 years for achieving the MDGs. All actors—government agencies, education and training institutions, professional associations, nongovernmental bodies, and private initiatives—should direct their efforts at a three-part agenda.

- Strengthening sustainable health systems in all countries.
- Mobilizing to combat health emergencies in crisis countries.
- Building the knowledge base for all.

For each part of the agenda, we set out the requirements and our specific recommendations (box 5.1).

Strengthening sustainable health systems

Every country, poor or rich, should have a national workforce plan to build sustainable health systems for addressing national health needs. These plans should aim to ensure access of every family to a motivated, skilled, and supported health worker. The skill mix, functions, and educational preparation of frontline workers should be shaped according to health needs and available resources. To optimize health system performance, where feasible, workers should be recruited from, accountable to, and supported for work in the community. Our specific recommendations:

Engaging stakeholders in planning and implementation should be at the heart of developing a national workforce strategic plan to guide investments in human resources and to strengthen the national health system.

- A national deliberative stakeholder process should assess, plan, design, and implement country workforce strategies.
- Although the consultative arrangements will vary by country, all should engage

> **Leaders of professional and training institutions should work closely with health policymakers to close the gap between the needs of health systems and the attitudes and skills imparted in education and training**

Box 5.1 | Key recommendations

Country-led and country-based strategies are the most important leverage points of all actions on human resources for health. We propose seven specific recommendations for country action backed by appropriate international reinforcement.

1. Every country should develop a national workforce strategic plan to guide enhanced investments in human resources aimed at strengthening the national health system. The plan should engage leaders and stakeholders, bring together health, education, finance, and other ministries, and ensure a positive policy environment.

2. Sub-Saharan African countries should retain workers in productive work environments and mobilize an additional 1 million workers, tripling the current numbers, to approach the MDGs.

3. All countries should develop core technical capacity in human resource strategic planning and management. International arrangements—pooled, virtual, or collaborative—should assemble country, regional, and global technical expertise to disseminate best practices and offer technical support to all countries.

4. Domestic and international investments in human resources for health should be expanded. A global educational reinvestment fund, cofinanced by local and foreign funds, should be launched to accelerate educational production in poor countries.

5. Donors should increase the impact of their human resource investments by devoting at least 10 percent—or $400 million—of their $4 billion spending on human resources to strengthening national capacities. Of these country investments, 10 percent—or $40 million—should be earmarked for strengthening technical and policy cooperation at the regional and global levels.

6. International donors and categorical funds and programs, such as those for HIV/AIDS, should invest and operate within country plans by adopting best practices for strengthening, not fragmenting, a sustainable workforce in national health systems.

7. An independent, nongovernmental, time-limited Action & Learning Initiative should succeed the Joint Learning Initiative to advocate for improvements in human resources for health, to promote the sharing of learning, to catalyze joint problem-solving among stakeholders, and monitor progress.

---

the health ministry and include finance, education, labor, and the civil service, as well as academic leaders, professional associations, labor unions, nongovernmental organizations, and the private sector.

Bringing health and education together is critical for harmonizing the supply of and demand for health workers. Academic leaders of professional and technical training institutions should work closely with health policymakers to close the gap between the needs of health systems and the attitudes and skills imparted in education and training.

- Educational and professional leaders should be consulted on health reform priorities. That can help in developing appropriate curricula, faculty capabilities, and career tracks for graduates. Special emphasis should be accorded to building leadership, management, and entrepreneurship.

" Finance and health policymakers should work together to develop an enabling fiscal environment for workforce development consistent with their political commitments to the MDGs

- Longer term educational planning and practices can improve downstream health system performance. For example, action to recruit both students and workers from underserved, marginalized communities is more likely to produce workers willing and able to serve in these communities.

Developing and disseminating best technical practices holds enormous potential for improving workforce policies and programs.

- Every country should develop core strategic and technical capacities in human resources for health. That capacity should be based in government as well as in academia and nongovernmental organizations.
- Institutional arrangements should be developed to link country, regional, and global technical expertise. Pooled, virtual, and operational networks should be assembled to disseminate best practices and offer technical support to country-led and country-based actions.

Crafting an equitable migration regime is a shared responsibility of all people and states. The regime should recognize "exceptionalism" in medical migration by promoting the human right of free movement while protecting the health of vulnerable populations.

- Countries that train skilled workers but suffer from unplanned out-migration must improve retention, incentives, and productivity while stepping up their investments in training and education, with curricula oriented to national, not international, priorities.

- Importing countries should dampen recruitment from poor low-density countries that suffer from unplanned out-migration. All countries, including OECD countries, should strive to attain self-sufficiency in worker production to reduce chronic dependency on imported workers.
- A global educational reinvestment fund should be established, not as a "compensation payment" but a shared investment for the benefit of all. The fund would accelerate educational production in poor sending countries.
- Schemes to promote the "reverse flow" of workers from high to low density countries should be explored—including the engagement of diaspora communities, sustainable systems of volunteers in nongovernmental and faith-based organizations, exchange fellows in twinning arrangements, and workers on time-limited contracts. The costs and hazards of reverse flows should be carefully evaluated, with schemes expanded only if they are effective and appropriate.

Ensuring supportive financial and donor policies is important because building a quality workforce requires an investment approach that provides adequate, stable, and sustained financing.

- Finance ministries and international financial institutions should regard finance for the workforce as an investment in human assets, not simply as a recurring cost or as social consumption. Designated as an investment, workforce allocations should be tracked in national and donor accounts.

> **❝ Donors should optimize the impact of their investments by applying at least 10 percent of their estimated $4 billion spending on human resources for strengthening strategic capacities within countries**

Box 5.2 | High stakes, high leverage

Strategic planning and management of human resources can leverage about two-thirds of domestic health budgets and nearly half of development assistance in health.

Of about $57 billion in development assistance, health allocations now total about $10 billion. Of this amount, about $4 billion is spent on salary, allowances, training, education, fellowships, technical assistance, and capacity building.

Now imagine that every country had strong national capacity. The strategic planning and management of human resources would optimize the performance of health systems. This would require both domestic and international investments in national capacity strengthening:

- If only 10 percent of development assistance in human resources for health were devoted to leveraging performance, $400 million would be available for investing

in human resource capacity in low-income countries.

- If 10 percent of these country investments were devoted to supporting international programs, $40 million would be available for an action alliance to support country action.

The impact of these two investments would be huge because the performance of the entire health sector would be improved through the strategic planning and management of human resources.

- Finance and health policymakers should work together to develop an enabling fiscal environment for workforce development. International financial institutions—consistent with their political commitments to the MDGs—should review and, if necessary, revise macroeconomic policies to strengthen a workforce commensurate with national health and development priorities.
- Donors should optimize the impact of their human resource investments by applying at least 10 percent—or $400 million—of their estimated $4 billion spending on human resources for strengthening strategic human capacities within countries (box 5.2). Ten percent of these country investments—or $40 million—should be earmarked for strengthening technical and policy cooperation at the regional and global level.
- Donors should move toward policies that expand their financing for the health

workforce, especially harmonizing project and categorical funding to strengthen, not fragment, the workforce of health systems. Coherence is particularly important in allowances and special payments, short-term training, and short-term tasks and assignments. Donors should audit all their investments for the impact on human resources in national health systems.

Mobilizing to combat health emergencies

In crisis countries severely affected by HIV/AIDS, especially in much of sub-Saharan Africa, popular movements to mobilize health workers are urgently required to end the crisis of human survival. Crisis countries must reinvigorate and, in some cases, reconfigure their workforce to expand capacity through appropriate delegation of health functions to community-based auxiliary workers. Because many of these countries depend heavily on external financing, the support of donors, regional bodies,

> **Effective action, both urgent and sustained, requires solid information, reliable analyses, and a firm knowledge base**

and global organizations is critical. Our specific recommendations:

Mobilizing workers in productive environments is central to emergency action for many countries to urgently tackle health crises.

- To approach the MDGs, urgent mobilization is required to triple the effective health workforce in sub-Saharan Africa (by an additional 1 million workers).
- The mobilization of new workers must be accompanied by strategies to retain current workers, to attract departed workers, and to create a productive work environment for all workers. Compensation and nonfinancial incentives should be planned and managed, and workers should be fully supported by ensuring drugs, supplies and equipment, supervision and training, and effective team support.
- In many countries, mobilization will be focused around combating such priority diseases as HIV/AIDS. While such categorical programs address high priority problems, workforce strategies should aim to steadily build health systems.

Strengthening, not fragmenting, health systems should be a principal objective of all programs, especially categorical programs focused on priority diseases.

- International donors and categorical funds and programs, such as those for HIV/AIDS, should invest and operate within country plans by adopting best practices for strengthening, not fragmenting, the health workforce.

- The dangers of fragmentation are especially high in low-income countries dependent on external resources, which are increasingly segmented into disease-specific efforts. These vertical efforts, for the longer term sustainability of their objectives, must build coherence into the development of human resources for stronger health systems.

Treating the need for additional human resources as an exception to address health emergencies is necessary in some crisis countries. To reverse health crises, some countries should consider exceptional macroeconomic policies, unusual measures to retain workers, and other emergency actions.

- Urgently create positive macroeconomic policies to build a workforce that can tackle the health emergency.
- Introduce special measures, as necessary, to retain a productive workforce, including exceptional organizational arrangements within or outside the civil service.

Building the knowledge base

Effective action, both urgent and sustained, requires solid information, reliable analyses, and a firm knowledge base. But data, analyses, and research on human resources for health and technical expertise are underdeveloped, in part due to chronic underinvestment. National and global learning processes must be launched to rapidly build the knowledge base—essential for guiding, accelerating, and improving action. A culture of science-based knowledge building must be infused into the human resources community. Our specific recommendations:

❝ We must spark a virtuous circle of acting, learning, adjusting, and growing

Collecting basic information and data should be undertaken by all countries, backed by the international system.

- All workers should be counted, and their social attributes and work functions should be collated. Trends and changes over time should be tracked.
- The global health metrics network should make human resources indicators a priority in essential health data.
- WHO should fulfill its core responsibility for maintaining comprehensive global statistical systems—adopting standard definitions and collecting robust information on human resources. The *World Health Report 2006* should sensitize the global health community to the importance of information and analysis for the health workforce.

Establishing norms, standards, and good practices is a critical knowledge function that can benefit workforce development in all countries.

- Research on workforce norms, standards, and best practices should be augmented, with the findings rapidly disseminated to improve workforce effectiveness in all countries.
- Learning networks and centers of technical excellence on workforce development, leadership, and management should be developed to enable the diffusion of best practices to all countries.

Building research and institutions for knowledge generation is central to the long-term development of human resources for health.

- Research programs in universities and institutes should be expanded to include labor economics, migration, management, educational methods, and other aspects of workforce development.
- Donors should significantly enhance their financing of research and information-gathering on human resources for health.

Completing an unfinished agenda: Action and learning

Implementing this work agenda demands immediate action backed by simultaneous learning. We must spark a virtuous circle of acting, learning, adjusting, and growing—because we do not have all the answers, and yet we must act urgently.

Because the key actions rest with national governments, we call on national leaders to implement these recommendations. Such leaders can come from both government and civil society, for both political and technical work.

Rather than launching yet another new global program, we call on existing international institutions to exercise their roles in supporting coherent national action. The value added by global action among existing organizations can be systematically strengthened so that international actors are more effective in supporting human resources for health strategies and actions at the country and community levels. The yardstick for the value added of international and global action is how well these activities support national action. Advocacy, technical cooperation, research and learning, and policy development are among some of the key functions. Existing organizations should focus on their comparative roles and capabilities,

" **All organizations must be held accountable for the coherence and implementation of their policy commitments**

strengthening collaboration and avoiding unproductive competition. All organizations must be held accountable for the coherence and implementation of their policy commitments. The following areas of comparative strength should be built on:

- The WHO should play a strong normative and technical leadership role, and the World Bank should incorporate human resource investment in its country-based concessional loans and grants while working with IMF to ensure enabling macroeconomic policies.
- Categorical funds and programs—such as Global Fund, the U.S. President's Emergency Plan for AIDS Relief, the Global Alliance on Vaccines and Immunizations, and other special programs to fight tuberculosis, malaria, polio, and measles and to improve maternal and child health—should develop explicit strategies to achieve their disease control targets while building a sustainable workforce.
- Regional bodies—such as the African Union, the New Partnership for Africa's Development, the Association of Southeast Asian Nations, the WHO Regional Office for Africa, and the Pan-American Health Organization—should advance human resources for health, especially through regional cooperation, educational collaboration, and the pooling of capabilities.
- The contributions of academic bodies, professional councils and associations, labor unions, and nongovernmental organizations should be promoted.

We propose also an independent, nongovernmental, five-year Action & Learning Initiative to succeed the Joint Learning Initiative (box 5.3).

Box 5.3 | Action & Learning Initiative

We propose an Action & Learning Initiative to undertake advocacy, link key actors, and conduct monitoring. Limited to five years and governed by global health leaders, the Initiative will have a focused work agenda, performing functions that existing organizations will not or cannot adequately take up.

Advocacy
- Promote political commitment, new financing, and public awareness
- Encourage and support performance of all existing actors

Linking actors
- Promote country leadership, the exchange of experiences, and problem solving
- Convene open biennial global forums

Monitoring
- Monitor policies, financing, and implementation of the JLI's recommendations
- Operate as clearinghouse for information

The Action & Learning Initiative will advocate for improvements in human resources for health, promote the sharing of learning, catalyze joint problem-solving by stakeholders, and monitor progress on the commitments of global organizations and country leaders. Operating through networks, with nodes in the major world regions, the Initiative will perform functions that existing organizations are either unwilling or unable to perform. A high priority will be accorded to engaging nongovernmental academic, professional, and social organizations.

The informal alliance for action can enhance the work of existing organizations and expand

At stake is nothing less than completing the 'unfinished health agenda' of the last century while addressing the unprecedented health challenges of this new century

the participation of fresh actors. The advantage of an alliance is that most critical activities can be conducted by existing organizations without creating yet another cumbersome and expensive global program or partnership. Success will depend, however, on how well existing institutions can ratchet up their capabilities and performance, and many will need significant donor support. Official agencies are urged to assume leadership roles in their respective areas of strength, even as the participation of nongovernmental groups is encouraged.

It is impossible to underestimate the importance of a response to this call for action. At stake is nothing less than completing the "unfinished health agenda" of the last century while addressing the unprecedented health challenges of this new century. Millions of people around the world are trapped in a vicious spiral of sickness and death. For them, there is no tomorrow without action today. Yet much can be done through rapidly mobilizing the workforce and wisely investing to build a stronger human infrastructure for sustainable health systems. What we do—or fail to do—will shape the course of global health in the 21st century.

Glossary

Unless otherwise noted, all definitions are drawn from the World Bank, the WHO, and Joint Learning Initiative Working Groups.

Accreditation   Approval of an institution or educational program by an authoritative government or professional body

Balance   Effective deployment and distribution of health personnel by geography, among levels of care, and among types of services for the equitable provision of quality health services

Brain drain   Outflow of health professionals to other countries, from the public to the private sector, or out of the health sector

Capacity building   Continuing process of strengthening individuals, groups, institutions, or societies to enhance their ability to perform core functions, to solve problems, and to achieve objectives

Civil society   Full scope of associational and civic practices that comprise activities of a society, separate from state and market institutions. Civil society includes nongovernmental organizations, religious institutions, foundations, guilds, professional associations, labor unions, academic institutions, media, public interest groups, and political parties

Competencies   Knowledge, skills, and attitudes that an individual accumulates, develops, and acquires through education, training, and work experiences

Complex adaptive systems   A complex, nonlinear, interactive system which adapts to a changing environment

Continuing professional development   Process of systematic learning that allows health professionals to update and enhance their skills and address their career and educational aspirations, while continuing to meet the needs of the population they serve

Cost-effectiveness   A measure of the comparative efficiency of discrete strategies and methods for achieving the same objective

Cultural factors   Customs, values, and norms of societies which affect health system dynamics, including gender, language, and residence

Deployment   Process of assigning personnel among regions or types and levels of services

Education   Preparing students for practice in the health system by equipping them with knowledge and skills, usually within established structures like medicine, nursing, and dentistry schools

Effectiveness   Producing services that are successful in preventing or treating disease and promoting health

Efficiency   Producing the maximum amount of health care with a fixed amount of resources

Employment   Condition in which personnel available for work in a labor market are utilized. Employment can be full-time or part-time, permanent or fixed-term

Equity   Fairness in the allocation of resources or outcomes among individuals or groups

Gender   Socially defined aspects and relationships related to being male or female

Ghost worker   Personnel formally on payroll but either absent or providing no service

Globalization   Increasing interconnectedness of countries through cross-border flows of goods, services, money, people, information, and ideas

Health planning   Planning for the optimal use of available resources for improvement of health services or health status over a given period

Health policies   A formal government statement or procedure, enacted through legislation or other forms of rule-making, which defines priorities and the parameters for action in response to health needs, available resources, and political perspectives

Health sector   The totality of policies, programs, and stakeholders, both governmental and private, which play a role in efforts aimed at improving people's health status

Health system   All activities whose primary purpose is to promote, restore, or maintain health

Heavily Indebted Poor Countries Initiative   An initiative launched by the World Bank and the IMF to help severely indebted countries reduce debt as part of an overall poverty reduction strategy

Human resources for health   All individuals engaged in the promotion, protection, or improvement of population health, from both the formal and informal sector

Human resource policies   Guidelines and directions within the health sector and the wider economic, social, and political context that regulate the use of workers

Imbalance   Shortage or surplus of health personnel as a result of disequilibrium between demand and supply for labor. Disparities in worker profession or specialty, geographic location, institutional facility, public or private allocation, and gender representation all cause imbalances

Incentives   Financial and nonfinancial benefits designed to improve staff performance and motivation

Innovation   The translation of ideas into new or improved services, processes, or systems

Knowledge management   The collection of processes that govern gathering, organizing, and disseminating intellectual and knowledge-based assets

Labor demand   The amount of services individuals or organizations would like to purchase from providers at current prices and wages. Health labor demand is conceptually different than the amount of provider services that is actually "needed" to improve population health

Labor market   Institutions and processes affecting the supply and demand for labor, through which employment and wages are determined

Labor supply   The amount of services health care professionals are willing to provide at current wages. Common measures of health labor supply include the number of providers per capita and total hours worked per provider

Licensing   Governmental authorization of a person to engage in a health occupation

Management   Process of creating an appropriate organizational environment and ensuring that personnel perform adequately using strategies to identify and achieve the optimal number, mix, and distribution of personnel in a cost-effective manner

Medium-term expenditure framework (MTEF)   A framework that reconciles estimates of aggregate resources available for public expenditure consistent with macroeconomic stability with estimates of the cost of carrying out policies (Source: www.undp.org.vn/projects/vie96028/whatis.pdf)

Mobility   The capacity for movement of personnel between positions, organizations, and regions

Motivation   An individuals' degree of willingness to sustain efforts towards achieving certain goals

Nongovernmental organization (NGO)   Private organizations that pursue activities to relieve suffering, promote the interests of the poor, provide basic social services, or undertake community development

Official development assistance (ODA)   Grants or loans to developing countries which are undertaken by the official sector at concessional financial terms with promotion of economic development and welfare as the main objective (Source: www.oecd.org)

Poverty reduction strategy paper (PRSP)   The basis for assistance from the World Bank and the International Monetary Fund as well as debt relief under the HIPC Initiative. PRSPs should be country-driven, comprehensive in scope, partnership-oriented, and participatory (Source: Commission on Macroeconomics and Health).

Private sector   In health care delivery, the private sector refers to nongovernment ownership or control and includes for-profit and nonprofit agencies

Productivity   Outputs extracted from given inputs, such as patients seen per worker or number of procedures per provider

Public health   Activities that protect the health of whole populations, such as the prevention of infectious disease, the reduction of contamination caused by private or commercial activities, and the regulation of workplace safety

Public sector   In health care delivery, the public sector refers to the government or agencies of the state

Recruitment   Process of searching for personnel to enter a particular job or position

Registration   Official recording of the names of persons who have certain qualifications to practice a profession or occupation

Remuneration   Payment to a person for a service or expense

Retention   Maintaining personnel within the health system, often by offering adequate incentives

Sector-wide approach (SWAp)   A strategy for development assistance in which a collective group of donor countries and a recipient country jointly plan, and commit to, a package of investments for a given sector (such as the health sector) (Source: Commision on Macroeconomics and Health)

Skill mix   The mix of posts, grades, or occupations in an organization. It may also refer to the combinations of activities or skills needed for each job within the organization

Stakeholders   Individuals or entities interested in, involved in, or potentially affected by a planned intervention, program, or project

Stock   Quantity of accumulated productive assets. With reference to the workforce, "stock" refers to the current composition of the workforce

Teamwork   Work done by a group formed by associates with different skills and backgrounds, with each doing a part to contribute to the efficiency of the whole

Training   Process of developing competencies in the provision of health care. Pre-service training takes place prior to employment, existing personnel benefit from in-service or on-the-job training

Unemployment   The condition in which personnel available for work in a labor market are not employed

Underemployment   The condition in which personnel available for full-time work in a labor market are employed at less than full-time or are in jobs where their full skills are not used

Union   Representative body of personnel that acts to protect and defend the legal rights and interests of their members, especially in issues involving conditions of pay, terms of employment, or job specifications

Vertical program   An approach to deliver health interventions for specific health problem(s), usually with explicit and well defined target(s) and a separate line of funding

Work environment   Characteristics of the environment in which a person is expected to work. Includes terms of employment, benefits, and physical and social climate

Workforce   People who work in the various professions of health care—physicians, nurses, midwives, pharmacists, dentists, associate professionals, and community health workers—whose goal is to improve the health of the populations they serve

Workforce planning   Process to provide a framework for staffing decisionmaking based on a strategic plan, budgetary resources, and a set of desired workforce competencies. It incorporates an analysis of the present and future workforce and possible gaps and surpluses

Workload   The amount of work expected of or assigned to a specific position or individual

Quantitative Information

This technical appendix compiles and consolidates the latest available quantitative information on the global health workforce in 186 countries.[1] Four technical tables provide qualitative and summary data on the number of health workers, the number of medical and nursing schools, selected health indicators, and financing related to the workforce. The appendix also presents summary data from a study commissioned by the Joint Learning Initiative on the relationship between health worker density and health outcomes.

Country clusters

In the four tables, all 186 countries are grouped into five clusters based on national health worker density (the HRH index) and health outcome (under-five mortality). The data used for clustering are contained in tables A2.1 and A2.3. Cut-offs for clustering countries are arbitrarily selected at 2.5 and 5.0 health workers (doctors, nurses, and midwives) per 1,000 population. An under-five mortality of 100 deaths per 1,000 live births was used to separate the low density countries into two groups—low density countries with high mortality and low density countries with low mortality. An under-five mortality of 9 deaths per 1,000 live births was used to separate the high-density countries into two groups—those with high mortality and those with low mortality.

Using these cut-offs, five clusters of countries were produced. Due to the limitation on the reliability of health worker data, interpretation of country characteristics in any specific cluster should be treated with caution. Even so, the general characteristics of countries in five clusters are as follows:

1) Low-density-high-mortality countries—low health worker density (below 2.5 per 1,000 population) and high under-five mortality rate (from 100 per 1,000 live births and above). This cluster consists mainly of the world's lowest income countries.

2) Low-density countries—low health worker density (below 2.5 per 1,000 population) and low under-five mortality rate (below 100 per 1,000 live births).

3) Moderate-density countries—health worker density between 2.5 and 5.0 per 1,000 population.

4) High-density countries—high health worker density (above 5.0 per 1,000 population) and high under-five mortality rate (from 9 per 1,000 live births and above). This cluster consists of many transitional economies and health worker exporting countries.

5) High-density-low-mortality countries—high health worker density (above 5.0 per 1,000 population) and low under-five mortality rate (below 9 per 1,000 live births). This cluster consists mostly of countries in the OECD.

Within each cluster, the countries are listed in alphabetical order. Where applicable, cluster average and cluster aggregate values are presented at the bottom of each cluster. Global cumulative and global average numbers are also shown at the end of each table.

Global health workers

Table A2.1 presents the global distribution of selected health workers. Data are compiled from the database Estimates of Health Personnel: Physicians, Nurses, Midwives, Dentists, and Pharmacists produced by the WHO Department of Human Resources for Health (as of August 17, 2004). Because many countries are not able to provide data on all health workers, only five major cadres of health workers are enumerated—physicians, nurses, midwives, dentists, and pharmacists. All quantitative estimations of health worker stock and density in this report are based on this database. The date (calendar year) of the estimates is approximately 2000, although individual countries vary around this year. Even though major efforts have been made to ensure validity, reliability, and completeness, the information in this database should be considered "estimates."

These data are the latest available official statistics on health personnel that WHO Headquarters in Geneva receives from ministries of health through its six regional offices, often with the cooperation of national statistical bodies. Upon submission, the data are scrutinized, reviewed, and triangulated using such additional sources as national and international employment surveys, records from professional associations, and other publications. If significant inconsistencies or differences are observed, the data are returned to national authorities for validation and resubmission.

The database is regularly updated through an ongoing process of collecting and analyzing country information in WHO headquarters. WHO cautions users of the database that country differences in data coverage, quality, and definitions will impose limitations on data consistency and comparability. For example, some countries provide information only for public sector workers, excluding private workers. Other countries may enumerate only physicians and nurses, not other workers.[2]

For the classification of health workers, WHO recommends compliance and use, wherever possible, of the International Labour Organization (ILO) international standard classification of occupations (ISCO) at the most detailed level (4 digits) of structure and definition. However, this standardization is incomplete. Many countries continue to use national definitions and classifications, variability that is inherent in this database. The physician group including generalists and specialists is defined by educational and certification procedures of individual countries. The nurse group includes all types of nurses, and likewise for midwives. Due to the limitation that some countries do not differentiate between nurses and midwives, only combined figures for nurses and midwives are presented here. Note that traditional midwives are excluded from these statistics. Also excluded are other categories of health workers, especially community health workers, traditional practitioners, and informal workers.

The health worker density index (HRH index) is a composite index calculated by the JLI team. It combines density of physicians, nurses, and midwives per 1,000 population, with the aim of reflecting, however imperfectly, the overall level of health workers in each country. As a significant number of missing values exist in the cases of dentist and pharmacist, these two professional groups are excluded from the HRH index. The HRH index is marked with a symbol if the combined nurses and midwives figure is missing; there is no missing value for physician numbers. No projection or estimation was done for missing values.

The HRH index is presented in every table in the appendix. In addition to health workers, the population size of each country is based on estimates of the UN Department of Economic and Social Affairs.[3] Information on geographical region as described by WHO's regional classification is also presented in the tables.

Global medical schools and nursing schools

Table A2.2 provides information on global medical and nursing education. It is recognized that health worker training is not limited to medical and nursing schools, but institutional data on public health schools, technical training institutes, health worker training centers, and other production facilities are unavailable. So this table provides data only on medical and nursing schools. In addition to these school statistics are selected education data that provide a broader contextual picture of education in the country.

Data on medical schools are from the Foundation for Advancement of International Medical Education and Research (FAIMER) based on its latest International Medical Education Directory, dated May 12, 2004. This directory contains a list of medical schools as provided by the *WHO World Directory of Medical Schools* (seventh edition). Additional medical schools have been added as FAIMER regularly updates its database whenever a new medical school is listed in its applications for medical degree certification (for non-U.S. medical graduates). To gain inclusion in the FAIMER directory, the medical school must already have produced medical graduates and must be officially acknowledged by the ministry of health or ministry of education.

Data on the nursing schools are less comprehensive. The table draws information from two sources—the fourth edition of "Nursing in the World" by the

International Nursing Foundation of Japan (2000) and the Pan-American Health Organization's "La enfermería en la Región de las Américas: Enfermería en la búsqueda de la equidad, la eficiencia, la eficacia y la calidad. Plan de Acción 1996–2001" (1997).

In addition to medical and nursing schools, selected educational indicators for each country are included in the table. Adult literacy rate, percentage of primary school completion, and percentage of primary, secondary, and tertiary school gross enrollment in 2000 are statistics from the World Bank's *World Development Indicators 2004.* Data on educational financing—public spending on education as percentage of government expenditure and percentage of GDP for the latest year (1998–2000)—come from the UNDP's *Human Development Report 2003.*

Global health indicators

Table A2.3 presents selected health and development indicators from countries that have health workforce statistics. Health statistics include life expectancy at birth and maternal, infant, and under-five mortality rate as health outcome indicators and poverty level, female literacy rate, and the composite human development index to reflect the level of country's development.

The infant mortality rate is expressed in term of number of deaths among infants per 1,000 live births while the under-five mortality rate measures number of deaths among children under five per 1,000 live births. Infant mortality rates are from the WHO's "Infant and Under Five Mortality Rates by WHO Region, Year 2000." Under-five mortality rates are for 2001, taken from UNICEF's *The State of the World's Children 2003,* unless otherwise specified. The latest available data on the maternal mortality rate statistics are from the 1995 WHO, UNICEF, and UNFPA Estimates of Maternal Mortality. They capture the number of maternal deaths per 100,000 live-births.

Poverty level indicates the proportion of population that live below one international PPP dollar per day as provided by the World Bank's *World Development Indicators 2003.* Latest available data were used so the years vary from 1993 to 2001. The WDI also provides statistics on life expectancy at birth for each country, for which the 2000 data are presented here.

A country's female adult literacy rate and human development index (HDI) for 2001 come from the UNDP *Human Development Report 2003.* Female adult literacy rate measures the proportion of female population above age 15 who are literate. The HDI is a composite index that summarizes a country's level of longevity, literacy and education, and standard of living. These are measured by life expectancy at birth, GDP per capita, adult literacy rate, and combined primary, secondary, and tertiary school enrollment ratios.

Global health workforce financing

Table A2.4 shows a country's income and its spending on health and the health workforce. Data on a country's income per capita come from the

WDI's gross national income and reflects the 2001 level in international dollars (based on purchasing power parity). Health spending per capita in the same year came from WHO National Health Accounts exercise as presented in the annex tables 5 and 6 of *World Health Report 2004*. Data are presented in U.S. dollars (at average exchange rates) and in international dollars.

The amount of official development assistance (ODA) for health received by countries as external resources is also from the WHO National Health Accounts. It is presented both in percentages of total health expenditure and in U.S. dollars. The estimated amount of ODA allocated to human resources for health is presented as a range of upper and lower bounds taken from the OECD Development Assistance Committee Database on Aid Activities. These upper and lower bounds are derived from available empirical evidence for bilateral agencies, which indicates that all bilateral agencies combined allocated between 28 and 41 percent of their three-year average commitments to the health sector between 1995 and 2002. These are likely to be underestimates as a result of the aggregated coding used in the database, which does not include a specific code for human resources. So, 30 percent and 50 percent are reasonably plausible lower and upper bounds that were used for the estimation exercise.

Human resources and health outcomes

As part of the JLI's research, a study was conducted to evaluate the variation between health worker density patterns and health outcomes. The full results of this study are presented in Anand and Baernighausen (2004). The objective of the cross-country regressions is to examine the relationship between health outcomes and human resources for health after controlling for the main socioeconomic determinants of health.

The total number of physicians, nurses, and midwives per population is chosen as a measure of health worker density. This aggregate measure is chosen, because the three categories of health care workers constitute the most-skilled health care personnel in most countries. Unfortunately, other important workers like community health workers were excluded because no comprehensive cross-country data set on their densities is available.

Per capita income (GNI PPP) is included as a first covariate. It serves as a general resources variable which captures the influence of several factors that influence mortality rates—including nutrition, safe water, sanitation, and housing.

Female adult literacy (FEMLIT) (proxying for female education) is included as a second covariate, because it is known to influence health through a variety of mechanisms, such as access, behavior, and lifestyle choices.

Absolute income poverty (INCPOV) is added as a covariate to take into account that with the same per capita income a higher rate of poverty would be expected to lead to higher mortality rates.

All dependent and independent variables are logarithmically transformed to reduce the number of outliers and to allow comparison with similar analyses. The data sources and variable definitions are given in the foregoing, except for the under-five mortality rate.[5]

Results

Human resources for health have a positive effect on mortality rates over and above the effects of income, education and poverty levels across countries: in all six regression equations, human resources for health are highly significant in explaining the maternal mortality rate, infant mortality rate, and under-five mortality rate, after controlling for the covariates (all $p < 0.001$).

The HRH elasticities of the different mortality rates range from −0.212 to −0.474, or a 10 percent increase in the number of HRH per population leads to a 2 to 5 percent decrease in the mortality rates. The HRH elasticity of the maternal mortality rate is higher than the HRH elasticities of infant mortality rate and under-five mortality rate. This finding is plausible: the impact of human resources for health is expected to be greater in averting maternal mortality than infant or child mortality because qualified medical personnel are able to address a larger proportion of conditions which put mothers at immediate risk of death compared with infants or children. The higher HRH elasticity of under-five mortality rate than of infant mortality rate observed may be the result of similar considerations: infants may face fewer medical conditions that put them at risk of death than children between one and four years of age, because infants may be relatively better protected by breastfeeding and other behaviors of mothers.

The coefficients of all covariates have the expected signs; the sizes of the coefficients are similar to those found in other studies of the determinants of maternal, infant, and under-five mortality.

Multiple regression equations with human resources for health as independent variable

Dependent variable	Regressions without income poverty			Regressions with income poverty		
	Maternal mortality (natural log)	Infant mortality (natural log)	Under-five mortality (natural log)	Maternal mortality (natural log)	Infant mortality (natural log)	Under-five mortality (natural log)
Independent variables						
Ln HRH	−0.474[b]	−0.235[b]	−0.260[b]	−0.474[b]	−0.212[b]	−0.231[b]
	(−5.182)	(−3.958)	(−4.154)	(−4.858)	(−2.998)	(−3.080)
Ln GNIPPP	−0.881[b]	−0.710[b]	−0.741[b]	−0.558[b]	−0.570[b]	−0.583[b]
	(−8.504)	(−10.539)	(−10.466)	(−4.022)	(−5.657)	(−5.461)
Ln FEMLIT	−0.304	−0.258[a]	−0.277[a]	−0.313	−0.273	−0.286
	(−1.327)	(−1.731)	(−1.767)	(−1.342)	(−1.613)	(−1.595)
Ln INCPOV				0.167[a]	0.106[a]	0.132[a]
				(1.899)	(1.666)	(1.950)
Constant	14.978[b]	11.183[b]	10.274[b]	12.071[b]	9.809[b]	8.653[b]
	(16.810)	(19.295)	(16.862)	(9.915)	(11.093)	(9.237)
N	117	117	117	83	83	83
R^2	0.791	0.815	0.818	0.791	0.787	0.789
F – statistics	142.535[b]	165.988[b]	169.008[b]	73.644[b]	71.882[b]	73.133

Note: The table shows regression coefficients with t-statistics in parentheses.

a. $p < 0.10$ b. $p < 0.01$

Ln HRH = Health worker density per population (natural log).

Ln GNIPPP = Per capita income (natural log).

Ln FEMLIT = Female adult literacy (natural log).

Ln INCPOV = Absolute income poverty (natural log).

N = Number of observations (countries).

Notes

1. Only 186 countries were included in the clustering exercise based on the availability of data for health worker density and under-five mortality.
2. More detailed explanation of the database, certain limitations, and the latest database version are accessible at the WHO Global Atlas of Health Workforce Website (www.who.int/globalatlas/autologin/hrh_login).
3. UN DESA 2004.
4. Available at www.oecd.org/dac/stats/crs/.
5. In these regressions, under-five mortality rate data is from the WHO for the year 2000 (www.who.int/child-adolescent-health/overview/child_health/mortality_rates_00.pdf).

References

Anand, Sudhir, and Till Baernighausen. 2004. "Human Resources and Health Outcomes: Cross-Country Econometric Study." *The Lancet* 364 (9445): 1603–9.

FAIMER (Foundation for Advancement of International Medical Education and Research). 2004. "International Medical Education Directory." [http://imed.ecfmg.org/main.asp].

International Nursing Foundation of Japan. 2000. *Nursing in the World: The Facts, Needs and Prospects*. Tokyo.

OECD (Organisation for Economic Co-operation and Development), Development Assistance Committee. "Database on Aid Activities." [www.oecd.org/dac/stats/crs/].

PAHO (Pan-American Health Organization). "La enfermería en la búsqueda de la equidad, la eficiencia, la eficacia y la calidad: Plan de Acción 1996–2001." Washington, D.C.

UN DESA (United Nations Department of Economic and Social Affairs). 2004. "Population Total, Estimates, and Projections, 2004." [http://unstats.un.org/unsd/].

UNDP (United Nations Development Programme). 2003. *Human Development Report 2003: Millennium Development Goals—A Compact Among Nations to End Human Poverty.* New York: Oxford University Press.

UNICEF (United Nations Children's Fund). 2003. *The State of the World's Children 2003.* [www.unicef.org/sowc03/contents/pdf/tables.pdf].

World Bank. 2003. *World Development Indicators 2003.* Washington, D.C.

———. 2004. *World Development Indicators 2004.* Washington, D.C.

World Health Organization. 1998. "Estimates of Health Personnel: Physicians, Nurses, Midwives, Dentists, and Pharmacists." [http://www3.who.int/whosis/health_personnel/health_personnel.cfm].

———. 2000a. "Infant and Under-Five Mortality Rates by WHO Region, Year 2000." [Retrieved October 8, 2004, from www.who.int/child-adolescent-health/OVERVIEW/CHILD_HEALTH/Mortality_Rates_00.pdf].

———. 2000b. *World Directory of Medical Schools.* 7th edition. Geneva.

———. 2004. *World Health Report 2004.* Geneva.

Table A2.1 Global distribution of health personnel

	Year	HRH Density	Physicians Number	Physicians Density	Nurses and midwives Number	Nurses and midwives Density	Dentists Number	Dentists Density	Pharmacists Number	Pharmacists Density	Population (thousands)	Region (WHO)	Source
Low-density-high-mortality													
Afghanistan	2001	0.40	4,104	0.19	4,752	0.22	630	0.03[a]	525	0.03[a]	22,083	EMR	Others
Angola	1997	1.27	881	0.08	13,598	1.19			24	0.00	11,447	AFR	HFA_africa
Benin	1995	0.34	315	0.06	1,548	0.28	16	0.00	154	0.03	5,470	AFR	HFA_africa
Burkina Faso	2001	0.34	490	0.04	3,666	0.30	36	0.00	60	0.01	12,259	AFR	MOH
Burundi	2000	0.34	323	0.05	1,783	0.28			62	0.01	6,267	AFR	MOH
Cambodia	2000	1.00	2,047	0.16	11,125	0.85	209	0.02	564	0.04	13,147	WPR	Others
Cameroon	1996	0.45	1,019	0.07	5,121	0.37	55	0.00			13,766	AFR	HFA_africa
Central African Republic	1995	0.17	117	0.04	459	0.14	7	0.00	26	0.01	3,354	AFR	HFA_africa
Chad	2001	0.20	205	0.03	1,381	0.17	2	0.00	38	0.01	8,103	AFR	Stat
Congo, Dem. Rep.	1996	0.51	3,129	0.07	20,046	0.44	499	0.01	907	0.02	45,353	AFR	HFA_africa
Congo, Rep.	1995	2.35	737	0.25	6,165	2.10					2,936	AFR	HFA_africa
Côte d'Ivoire	1996	0.55	1,322	0.09	6,785	0.46					14,685	AFR	HFA_africa
Djibouti	1999	0.79	86	0.13	424	0.65	10	0.02	12	0.02	648	EMR	Others
Equatorial Guinea	1996	0.67	101	0.25	171	0.42	4	0.01	8	0.02	411	AFR	HFA_africa
Eritrea	1996	0.21	98	0.03	595	0.18	3	0.00	16	0.01	3,271	AFR	HFA_africa
Ethiopia	2002	0.23	1,971	0.03	14,160	0.21	61	0.00	125	0.00	68,961	AFR	MOH
Gambia, The	1997	0.25	42	0.04	247	0.21	6	0.01	6	0.01	1,193	AFR	HFA_africa
Ghana	2002	0.93	1,842	0.09	17,196	0.84	36	0.00[b]	1,433	0.07	20,471	AFR	MOH
Guinea	2000	0.56	764	0.09	3,805	0.47	38	0.01	199	0.02	8,117	AFR	Others
Guinea-Bissau	1996	1.39	203	0.17	1,496	1.22	11	0.01	12	0.01	1,225	AFR	HFA_africa
Haiti	1998	0.36	1,949	0.25	834	0.11	94	0.01			7,797	AMR	Others
Kenya	1995	1.03	3,616	0.13	24,679	0.90	603	0.02	1,370	0.05	27,390	AFR	HFA_africa
Lao PDR	1996	1.62	2,812	0.59	4,931	1.03	196	0.04			4,801	WPR	Others
Lesotho	1995	1.12	91	0.05	1,802	1.07	8	0.01	17	0.01	1,683	AFR	HFA_africa
Liberia	1997	0.12	55	0.02	244	0.10	2	0.00			2,395	AFR	HFA_africa
Madagascar	2001	0.36	1,428	0.09	4,560	0.28	76	0.01	8	0.00	16,439	AFR	MOH
Malawi	2003	0.31	599	0.05	3,094	0.26	4	0.00	39	0.00	12,105	AFR	Others
Mali	2000	0.19	529	0.04	1,785	0.15	10	0.00[c]			11,904	AFR	Stat
Mauritania	1995	0.86	317	0.14	1,667	0.72	46	0.02	95	0.04	2,300	AFR	HFA_africa
Mozambique	2000	0.31	435	0.02	5,078	0.28	136	0.01	419	0.02	17,861	AFR	MOH
Myanmar	2000	0.78	14,356	0.30	22,949	0.48	984	0.02[a]			47,545	SEAR	MOH
Niger	2002	0.30	386	0.03	3,129	0.27	21	0.00	63	0.01	11,544	AFR	Others
Nigeria	2000	1.45	30,885	0.27	108,203	1.19[d]	2,180	0.02	8,642	0.08	114,746	AFR	MOH
Pakistan	2001	1.13	96,900	0.66	68,400	0.47	4,560	0.03	45,390	0.31	146,277	EMR	Others
Rwanda	2002	0.23	155	0.02	1,745	0.21	4	0.00	11	0.00	8,273	AFR	MOH
Senegal	1995	0.36	625	0.08	2,393	0.29	100	0.01	225	0.03	8,338	AFR	HFA_africa
Sierra Leone	1996	0.45	300	0.07	1,548	0.38	16	0.00			4,105	AFR	HFA_africa
Somalia	1997	0.23	310	0.04	1,486	0.19	15	0.00	8	0.00	7,763	EMR	Others

Table A2.1 Global distribution of health personnel (continued)

	Year	HRH Density	Physicians Number	Physicians Density	Nurses and midwives Number	Nurses and midwives Density	Dentists Number	Dentists Density	Pharmacists Number	Pharmacists Density	Population (thousands)	Region (WHO)	Source
Low-density-high-mortality													
Sudan	2000	1.01	4,973	0.16	26,730	0.85	218	0.01	311	0.01	31,437	EMR	Others
Tanzania	2002	0.39	822	0.02	13,292	0.37	216	0.01[e]	365	0.01	36,276	AFR	MOH
Togo	2001	0.30	265	0.06	1,128	0.24	25	0.01	141	0.03	4,686	AFR	MOH
Uganda	2002	0.14	1,175	0.05	2,200	0.09	75	0.00	125	0.01	25,004	AFR	MOH
Yemen, Rep.	2001	0.67	4,078	0.22	8,342	0.45	222	0.01	1,237	0.07[a]	18,651	EMR	Others
Zambia	1995	1.20	647	0.07	10,598	1.13	122	0.01	75	0.01	9,371	AFR	HFA_africa
Zimbabwe	2002	0.60	736	0.06	6,951	0.54	15	0.00	12	0.00	12,835	AFR	MOH
Cluster cumulative			**188,240**		**442,291**		**11,571**		**62,724**		**855,000**		
Cluster weighted average		**0.77**	**22,692**	**0.22**	**34,177**	**0.55**	**1,288**	**0.01**	**10,517**	**0.08**	**60,000**		
Low-density													
Bangladesh	2001	0.47	32,498	0.23	33,929	0.24					140,880	SEAR	Others
Belize	2000	2.31	251	1.05	303	1.26	32	0.13			240	AMR	Others
Bhutan	1999	0.28	103	0.05	467	0.23					2,004	SEAR	Others
Bolivia	2001	1.05	6,220	0.73	2,698	0.32	692	0.08			8,481	AMR	Others
Cape Verde	1996	0.73	68	0.17	222	0.56	6	0.02			400	AFR	HFA_africa
Chile	2003	1.72	17,250	1.09	10,000	0.63	6,750	0.43			15,806	AMR	Others
Colombia	2002	1.90	58,761	1.35	23,940	0.55	33,951	0.78			43,526	AMR	Others
Comoros	1997	0.55	48	0.07	310	0.48	90	0.14			646	AFR	HFA_africa
Costa Rica	2000	2.39	6,788	1.73	2,600	0.66	1,847	0.47			3,929	AMR	Others
El Salvador	2002	2.03	7,938	1.24	5,103	0.80	3,465	0.54			6,415	AMR	Others
Fiji	1999	2.30	271	0.34	1,576	1.96	32	0.04	59	0.07	805	WPR	Others
Gabon	1995	0.29	321	0.29							1,109	AFR	Stat
Honduras	1997	1.09	4,960	0.83	1,520	0.26	1,002	0.17			5,962	AMR	Others
India	1998	1.13	503,900	0.51	607,376	0.62					983,110	SEAR	Others
Indonesia	2000	0.65	34,347	0.16	103,918	0.49	2,406	0.01			211,559	SEAR	Stat
Malaysia	2000	2.39	16,146	0.70	38,840	1.69	2,144	0.09	2,333	0.10	23,001	WPR	MOH
Maldives	2000	2.01	226	0.78	358	1.23					291	SEAR	Others
Morocco	2001	1.48	14,293	0.48	29,462	1.00	2,304	0.08	4,901	0.17	29,585	EMR	Others
Nepal	2001	0.31	1,259	0.05	6,216	0.26					24,060	SEAR	MOH
Nicaragua	2003	1.78	8,986	1.64	765	0.14	1,585	0.29			5,466	AMR	Others
Papua New Guinea	2000	0.58	275	0.05	2,841	0.53	90	0.02			5,334	WPR	MOH
Paraguay	2000	1.37	6,400	1.17	1,089	0.20	1,947	0.36			5,470	AMR	Others
Peru	1999	1.84	29,799	1.17	17,108	0.67	2,809	0.11			25,535	AMR	Others
São Tomé and Principe	1996	2.04	63	0.47	211	1.57	7	0.05	2	0.01	134	AFR	HFA_africa
Solomon Islands	1999	0.98	54	0.13	361	0.85	26	0.06	28	0.07	424	WPR	Others
Sri Lanka	2000	1.22	7,963	0.43	14,716	0.79	461	0.03[a]	830	0.05[a]	18,595	SEAR	MOH

	Year	HRH Density	Physicians Number	Physicians Density	Nurses and midwives Number	Nurses and midwives Density	Dentists Number	Dentists Density	Pharmacists Number	Pharmacists Density	Population (thousands)	Region (WHO)	Source
Low-density													
Suriname	2000	2.07	191	0.45	688	1.62	4	0.01			425	AMR	Others
Thailand	1999	1.92	18,140	0.30	97,515	1.62					60,306	SEAR	MOH
Vanuatu	1997	2.46	20	0.11	428	2.35					182	WPR	Others
Vietnam	2001	1.28	42,327	0.53	59,201	0.75			5,977	0.08	79,197	WPR	Others
Cluster cumulative			**819,866**		**1,063,761**		**61,650**		**14,130**		**1,700,000**		
Cluster weighted average		**1.11**	**303,305**	**0.48**	**375,128**	**0.63**	**5,714**	**0.15**	**4,531**	**0.09**	**614,000**		
Moderate-density													
Algeria	1995	3.82	23,585	0.85	83,022	2.98	7,862	0.28	3,624	0.13	27,878	AFR	HFA_africa
Antigua and Barbuda	1999	3.45	12	0.17	233	3.28	13	0.18[f]			71	AMR	Others
Argentina	1998	3.81	108,800	3.00	29,000	0.80	28,900	0.80	15,300	0.42	36,153	AMR	Others
Barbados	1999	4.92	322	1.21	988	3.71	63	0.24			267	AMR	Others
Botswana	1999	2.70	488	0.29	4,090	2.41	38	0.02	142	0.08	1,697	AFR	MOH
Brazil	2001	2.57	357,888	2.06	89,710	0.52	165,599	0.95	66,727	0.38	174,029	AMR	Others
Brunei	2000	4.89	336	1.01	1,296	3.88	48	0.14	90	0.27	334	WPR	MOH
China	2002	2.68	2,122,019	1.64	1,345,706	1.04			368,852	0.29[a]	1,291,966	WPR	Stat
Dominica	1997	4.65	38	0.49	317	4.16	4	0.06			76	AMR	Others
Dominican Republic	2000	3.72	15,670	1.88	15,352	1.84	7,000	0.84	3,330	0.40	8,353	AMR	Others
Ecuador	2000	3.13	18,335	1.48	20,586	1.66	2,062	0.17			12,420	AMR	Others
Egypt, Arab Rep.	2000	4.88	143,555	2.12	187,017	2.76	18,438	0.27	46,096	0.68	67,784	EMR	Others
Grenada	1997	4.17	41	0.50	303	3.68	7	0.09			82	AMR	Others
Guatemala	1999	4.94	9,965	0.90	44,986	4.05	2,046	0.18			11,122	AMR	Others
Guyana	2000	2.77	366	0.48	1,738	2.29	30	0.04			759	AMR	Others
Iran, Islamic Rep.	1998	3.51	68,079	1.05	155,542	2.46[b]	12,378	0.19	8,108	0.13	64,887	EMR	Others
Iraq	2001	3.62	12,955	0.54	69,525	3.08[a]	2,689	0.11	1,955	0.08	23,861	EMR	Others
Jamaica	2003	2.50	2,253	0.85	4,374	1.65	212	0.08			2,651	AMR	Others
Jordan	2001	4.80	10,623	2.05	14,251	2.75	2,850	0.55	4,975	0.96	5,183	EMR	Others
Kiribati	1998	2.64	24	0.30	191	2.34	4	0.05	4	0.05	82	WPR	Others
Lebanon	2001	4.43	11,505	3.25	4,157	1.18	4,283	1.21	3,359	0.95	3,537	EMR	Others
Libya	1997	4.89	6,371	1.29	17,779	3.60	693	0.14	1,225	0.25	4,939	EMR	Others
Marshall Islands	2000	3.45	24	0.47	152	2.98	4	0.08	2	0.04	51	WPR	Others
Mauritius	1995	3.18	956	0.85	2,619	2.33	152	0.14	223	0.20	1,125	AFR	HFA_africa
Mexico	2001	3.93	172,266	1.71	222,389	2.21	9,669	0.01			100,456	AMR	Others
Micronesia, Fed. Sts.	2000	4.50	64	0.60	417	3.90	14	0.13			107	WPR	Others
Namibia	1997	3.14	516	0.30	4,978	2.84	70	0.04	149	0.09	1,750	AFR	HFA_africa
Oman	2002	4.23	3,478	1.26	8,004	2.98[g]	297	0.11[g]	594	0.22[g]	2,768	EMR	Others
Palau	1998	2.56	20	1.09	27	1.47	2	0.11	1	0.05	18	WPR	Others

	Year	HRH Density	Physicians Number	Physicians Density	Nurses and midwives Number	Nurses and midwives Density	Dentists Number	Dentists Density	Pharmacists Number	Pharmacists Density	Population (thousands)	Region (WHO)	Source
Moderate-density													
Panama	2000	3.20	4,942	1.68	4,484	1.52	1,421	0.48			2,950	AMR	Others
Samoa	1999	2.74	120	0.70	349	2.04	30	0.18	5	0.03	171	WPR	MOH
Saudi Arabia	2001	4.44	31,896	1.40	69,421	3.04	3,672	0.17[h]	5,420	0.24	22,829	EMR	Others
South Africa	2001	4.57	30,740	0.69	172,338	3.88	4,648	0.10	10,742	0.24	44,416	AFR	Others
St. Vincent and the Grenadines	1997	3.26	101	0.88	276	2.39	6	0.05			116	AMR	Others
Swaziland	2000	3.38	184	0.18	3,345	3.20	20	0.02	46	0.04	1,044	AFR	HFA_africa
Syrian Arab Republic	2001	3.34	23,742	1.40	32,938	1.94	12,206	0.72	8,862	0.52	16,968	EMR	Others
Tonga	2001	3.70	35	0.34	341	3.36	33	0.32	17	0.17	102	WPR	Others
Trinidad and Tobago	1997	3.66	1,004	0.79	3,653	2.87	107	0.08			1,274	AMR	Others
Tunisia	1997	3.57	6,459	0.70	26,389	2.87	1,200	0.13	1,569	0.17	9,193	EMR	Others
Turkey	2001	4.19	86,000	1.24	204,183	2.95	15,866	0.23	22,922	0.33	69,303	EUR	Others
Uruguay	2002	4.50	12,384	3.65	2,880	0.85	3,936	1.16			3,391	AMR	Others
Venezuela, RB	2001	2.58	48,000	1.94	15,020	0.64[f]	13,680	0.55			24,752	AMR	Others
Cluster cumulative			3,336,161		2,864,366		322,252		574,339		2,040,000		
Cluster weighted average		3.05	1,396,723	1.64	896,687	1.41	47,103	0.43	263,205	0.31	848,000		
High-density													
Albania	2000	5.43	4,325	1.39	12,570	4.04	1,390	0.45[i]	1,300	0.40[c]	3,113	EUR	Others
Armenia	2001	8.76	10,889	3.53	16,173	5.24	710	0.23	121	0.04	3,088	EUR	Others
Azerbaijan	2001	12.04	29,084	3.54	69,929	8.50	2,116	0.26	2,143	0.26	8,226	EUR	HFA_Europe
Bahamas, The	1998	5.53	312	1.06	1,323	4.47	21	0.07			296	AMR	Others
Bahrain	2001	5.72	1,106	1.60	2,861	4.13	144	0.21	151	0.22	693	EMR	Others
Belarus	2001	17.45	44,902	4.50	129,352	12.95	4,393	0.44	3,001	0.30	9,986	EUR	HFA_Europe
Bosnia and Herzegovina	2001	5.73	5,443	1.34	17,867	4.39	679	0.17	350	0.09	4,067	EUR	Others
Bulgaria	2001	8.26	27,186	3.38	39,139	4.87	6,482	0.81	1,020	0.13[h]	8,033	EUR	Others
Cuba	2002	13.35	66,567	5.91	83,880	7.44	9,841	0.87			11,271	AMR	MOH
Estonia	2001	9.78	4,275	3.16	8,956	6.62	1,094	0.81	813	0.59[h]	1,353	EUR	HFA_Europe
Georgia	2002	7.92	20,225	3.91	20,798	4.02	1,532	0.30	364	0.07	5,177	EUR	HFA_others
Hungary	2001	11.89	31,768	3.16[a]	86,983	8.73	4,618	0.46[a]	5,024	0.50	9,968	EUR	HFA_Europe
Kazakhstan	2001	9.50	51,289	3.30	96,234	6.20	4,337	0.28	2,672	0.17	15,533	EUR	Others
Korea, Dem. Rep.	1995	5.37	63,478	2.97	51,294	2.40					21,373	SEAR	Others
Kuwait	2001	5.43	3,589	1.53	9,197	3.91	673	0.29	722	0.32[h]	2,353	EMR	Others
Kyrgyz Republic	2001	10.05	13,379	2.68	36,838	7.38	1,077	0.22	109	0.02	4,995	EUR	HFA_Europe
Latvia	2001	8.21	6,851	2.91	12,455	5.30	1,245	0.53			2,351	EUR	HFA_Europe
Lithuania	2001	12.39	14,031	4.03	29,137	8.36	2,490	0.71	2,266	0.65	3,484	EUR	HFA_others
Macedonia, FYR	2001	8.09	4,459	2.19	12,009	5.90	1,125	0.55	309	0.15	2,035	EUR	HFA_Europe
Moldova	2001	9.21	11,520	2.69	27,840	6.51	1,326	0.31	2,621	0.61	4,276	EUR	Others

Table A2.1 Global distribution of health personnel (continued)

	Year	HRH Density	Physicians Number	Physicians Density	Nurses and midwives Number	Nurses and midwives Density	Dentists Number	Dentists Density	Pharmacists Number	Pharmacists Density	Population (thousands)	Region (WHO)	Source
High-density													
Mongolia	2002	5.95	6,823	2.67	8,414	3.29	469	0.18	788	0.31	2,559	WPR	MOH
Philippines	2002	7.37	91,408	1.16	488,024	6.21	44,129	0.56	47,463	0.60	78,580	WPR	Others
Poland	2000	7.67	85,031	2.20	211,629	5.47	11,758	0.30	22,161	0.57	38,671	EUR	Others
Qatar	2001	7.15	1,310	2.21	2,917	4.93	220	0.37	530	0.90	591	EMR	Others
Romania	2001	6.20	42,339	1.89	96,813	4.32	5,057	0.23	1,490	0.07	22,437	EUR	Others
Russian Federation	2001	12.51	604,365	4.17	1,207,873	8.34	46,209	0.32	10,215	0.07	144,877	EUR	Others
Seychelles	1996	9.95	100	1.32	653	8.62[a]	9	0.12	4	0.05	76	AFR	HFA_africa
Slovak Republic	2001	10.63	17,556	3.25	39,783	7.38	2,378	0.44	2,605	0.48	5,394	EUR	Others
St. Kitts and Nevis	1997	6.16	51	1.18	216	4.98	8	0.18			43	AMR	Others
St. Lucia	1999	7.47	749	5.18	331	2.29	9	0.06			145	AMR	Others
Tajikistan	2001	7.20	13,393	2.18	30,819	5.02	1,051	0.17	680	0.11	6,144	EUR	Others
Turkmenistan	1997	10.20	13,946	3.17	30,894	7.03	1,004	0.23	1,554	0.35	4,398	EUR	Others
Ukraine	2001	11.16	146,582	2.97	403,442	8.19	19,275	0.39			49,290	EUR	Others
United Arab Emirates	2001	6.21	5,825	2.02	12,045	4.18	954	0.33	1,086	0.38	2,879	EMR	Others
Uzbekistan	2001	13.67	73,041	2.89	273,114	10.79	5,283	0.21	673	0.03	25,313	EUR	HFA_Europe
Cluster cumulative			**1,517,197**		**3,571,802**		**183,106**		**112,235**		**503,000**		
Cluster weighted average		**10.12**	**224,289**	**3.02**	**513,736**	**7.10**	**25,379**	**0.38**	**15,123**	**0.27**	**66,800**		
High-density-low-mortality													
Andorra	2001	5.77	175	2.59	214	3.17	42	0.62	64	0.95	68	EUR	Others
Australia	2001	10.84	48,211	2.49	161,585	8.35	8,200	0.42	13,956	0.72	19,352	WPR	Others
Austria	2001	9.33	26,286	3.24	49,346	6.09	4,029	0.50	4,581	0.57	8,106	EUR	Others
Belgium	2001	15.58	42,978	4.18	115,798	11.39[b]	7,106	0.70[i]	14,772	1.45[i]	10,273	EUR	HFA_Europe
Canada	2000	12.20	64,454	2.09	311,091	10.11	17,287	0.56	24,518	0.80	30,770	AMR	Others
Croatia	2001	7.70	10,552	2.37	23,676	5.33	3,021	0.68	2,235	0.50	4,445	EUR	Others
Cyprus	2000	7.84	2,336	2.98	3,803	4.86	803	1.03	758	0.97	783	EMR	Others
Czech Republic	2001	13.38	35,222	3.43	101,972	9.94	6,698	0.65	5,199	0.51	10,257	EUR	HFA_others
Denmark	2002	13.62	19,600	3.66	53,302	9.96	4,834	0.90	2,638	0.49	5,351	EUR	Others
Finland	2001	25.59	16,110	3.11	116,617	22.48	4,731	0.91	7,755	1.50	5,188	EUR	HFA_others
France	2001	10.21	196,000	3.29	412,231	6.92	40,426	0.68	60,366	1.01	59,564	EUR	MOH
Germany	2001	13.24	297,893	3.62	792,506	9.62	63,854	0.78	47,692	0.58	82,349	EUR	Others
Greece	2001	7.50	47,944	4.40	32,449	3.10[e]	12,394	1.14			10,947	EUR	HFA_Europe
Iceland	2001	13.17	990	3.47	2,763	9.70	283	1.00[h]	243	0.85	285	EUR	HFA_Europe
Ireland	2001	18.99	9,166	2.37	63,474	16.62[h]	2,006	0.52	3,165	0.82	3,865	EUR	HFA_others
Israel	2001	10.25	24,140	3.91	39,137	6.34	7,387	1.20	4,176	0.68	6,174	EUR	Others
Italy	2001	10.53	348,862	6.07	256,860	4.46[a]	34,014	0.59	63,008	1.01	57,521	EUR	Others
Japan	2000	10.41	255,792	2.01	1,066,979	8.40	90,857	0.72	217,477	1.71	127,034	WPR	MOH

A2

	Year	HRH Density	Physicians Number	Physicians Density	Nurses and midwives Number	Nurses and midwives Density	Dentists Number	Dentists Density	Pharmacists Number	Pharmacists Density	Population (thousands)	Region (WHO)	Source
High-density-low-mortality													
Korea, Rep.	2000	5.42	84,611	1.81	169,029	3.61	18,039	0.39	50,623	1.08	46,836	WPR	Others
Luxembourg	2001	10.45	1,123	2.55	3,486	7.90	283	0.64	325	0.74	441	EUR	HFA_others
Malta	2001	6.69	1,144	2.93	1,473	3.77	158	0.40	750	1.92	391	EUR	Others
Monaco	1995	20.47	186	5.86	464	14.61	34	1.07	61	1.92	32	EUR	HFA_Europe
Netherlands	2001	16.73	52,602	3.29	214,853	13.44	7,509	0.47	3,148	0.20	15,983	EUR	HFA_Europe
New Zealand	2001	10.91	8,491	2.23	33,124	8.68	1,601	0.42	3,808	1.00	3,815	WPR	Council
Norway	2001	24.89	15,978	3.56	95,880	21.34	5,627	1.25	1,781	0.40	4,494	EUR	HFA_others
Portugal	2000	6.98	32,498	3.24	37,477	3.74	4,370	0.44	8,056	0.80	10,016	EUR	Others
San Marino	1990	7.85	58	2.52	123	5.34	8	0.36	12	0.52	23	EUR	HFA_Europe
Singapore	2001	5.64	5,747	1.40	17,398	4.24	1,087	0.26	1,141	0.28	4,105	WPR	Others
Slovenia	2001	9.36	4,361	2.19	14,245	7.17	1,178	0.59	776	0.39	1,988	EUR	HFA_Europe
Spain	2000	6.82	130,300	3.20	147,500	3.62	17,538	0.43	31,200	0.77	40,752	EUR	HFA_Europe
Sweden	2000	13.49	26,979	3.05	92,491	10.44			5,317	0.60	8,856	EUR	Others
Switzerland	2000	12.14	25,216	3.52	61,866	8.63	3,468	0.48	4,450	0.62	7,173	EUR	Others
United Kingdom	1993	7.06	95,395	1.66	309,379	5.40	23,100	0.40	33,760	0.59	57,309	EUR	Others
United States	2000	13.22	1,564,400	5.49	2,201,800	7.73	168,000	0.59	196,100	0.69	285,003	AMR	Others
Cluster cumulative			3,495,800		7,004,391		559,972		813,911		930,000		
Cluster weighted average		11.30	598,107	3.76	992,118	7.54	79,586	0.61	110,875	0.89	130,000		
Global cumulative			9,357,264		14,946,611		1,138,551		1,577,339		6,028,000		
Global minimum		0.12	12	0.02	27	0.09	2	0.00	1	0.00	18		
Global maximum		25.59	2,122,019	6.06	2,201,800	22.48	168,000	1.25	368,852	1.92	1,291,966		
Global weighted average		4.04	672,395	1.55	610,004	2.49	36,715	0.34	148,678	0.38	494,367		

a. Data are for 1999. b. Data are for 1996. c. Data are for 1994. d. Data are for 1992. e. Data are for 1995. f. Data are for 1997. g. Data are for 2001. h. Data are for 2000. i. Data are for 1998.

Table A2.2 Global distribution of medical schools and nursing schools

Country	Year	HRH density	Medical schools	Nursing schools	Adult literacy	Primary school Completion rate (%)	Primary school Enrollment (%)	Secondary school enrollment (%)	Tertiary school enrollment (%)	Public education expenditure Percent of GDP	Public education expenditure Percent of government expenditure
Low-density-high-mortality											
Afghanistan	2001	0.40	4				15				
Angola	1997	1.27	1			28		17		2.70	
Benin	1995	0.34	1		37	43	97			3.20	
Burkina Faso	2001	0.34	1			28	44	10			
Burundi	2000	0.34	1		48	27	66	10	1	3.40	
Cambodia	2000	1.00	1	5	68	56	111	18	2	1.90	10.10
Cameroon	1996	0.45	1		71	55	106		5	3.20	12.50
Central African Republic	1995	0.17	1		49	19	75			1.90	
Chad	2001	0.20	1		43	21	73			2.00	
Congo, Dem. Rep.	1996	0.51	3			40					
Congo, Rep.	1995	2.35	1		81	56	84		4	4.20	12.60
Côte d'Ivoire	1996	0.55	1			45	78			4.60	21.50
Djibouti	1999	0.79		1		33	40	18	1	3.50	
Equatorial Guinea	1996	0.67				49	130	29		0.60	
Eritrea	1996	0.21					57	27	2	4.80	
Ethiopia	2002	0.23	3		39	27	61	17	2	4.80	13.80
Gambia, The	1997	0.25				71	79	34		2.70	14.20
Ghana	2002	0.93	2	2	72	57	79	36	3	4.10	
Guinea	2000	0.56	1			34	67			1.90	25.60
Guinea-Bissau	1996	1.39	1			31				2.10	4.80
Haiti	1998	0.36	1	2	50					1.10	10.90
Kenya	1995	1.03	2	5	82	42	94	31	3	6.40	22.50
Lao PDR	1996	1.62	1	1	65	72	113	38	3	2.30	8.80
Lesotho	1995	1.12		1	83	64	122	32	3	10.10	18.50
Liberia	1997	0.12	1		54						
Madagascar	2001	0.36	2			35	103		2	3.20	10.20
Malawi	2003	0.31	1	1	60	53				4.10	24.60
Mali	2000	0.19	1		19	35	54			2.80	
Mauritania	1995	0.86			40	47	85	22	4	3.00	18.90
Mozambique	2000	0.31	1		44	38	91	12		2.40	12.30
Myanmar	2000	0.78	3	2	85	71	90	39	12	0.50	9.00
Niger	2002	0.30	1	2	16	20	36	7	2	2.70	
Nigeria	2000	1.45	15	3	64	67					
Pakistan	2001	1.13	19	65		55	73			1.80	7.80
Rwanda	2002	0.23	1		67	20	117	15	2	2.80	

Table A2.2 Global distribution of medical schools and nursing schools (continued)

Country	Year	HRH density	Medical schools	Nursing schools	Adult literacy	Primary school Completion rate (%)	Primary school Enrollment (%)	Secondary school enrollment (%)	Tertiary school enrollment (%)	Public education expenditure Percent of GDP	Public education expenditure Percent of government expenditure
Low-density-high-mortality											
Senegal	1995	0.36	1	1	37	46	74	17		3.20	
Sierra Leone	1996	0.45	1			32	79		2	1.00	
Somalia	1997	0.23	1								
Sudan	2000	1.01	14		58	50	58	32			
Tanzania	2002	0.39	2	1	75	49	64	6	1	2.10	
Togo	2001	0.30	1		57		123			4.80	23.20
Uganda	2002	0.14	3	1	67	61	134		3	2.30	
Yemen, Rep.	2001	0.67	2		46	65	79	46		10.00	32.80
Zambia	1995	1.20	1	1	78		79		2	2.30	17.60
Zimbabwe	2002	0.60		1	89		96	43	4	10.40	
Cluster cumulative			**99**	**95**							
Cluster weighted average		**0.77**	**7**	**21**	**61**	**50**	**77**	**24**	**4**	**3**	**13**
Low-density											
Bangladesh	2001	0.47	11	1	40	73	99	46	6	2.50	15.70
Belize	2000	2.31	2	1	77	87	118	71		6.20	20.90
Bhutan	1999	0.28		1		42				5.20	12.90
Bolivia	2001	1.05	10	11	85	82	115	80	37	5.50	23.10
Cape Verde	1996	0.73			74	95	123	66		4.40	
Chile	2003	1.72	6	12	96	91	103	86	37	4.20	17.50
Colombia	2002	1.90	26	27	92	89	112	70	23		
Comoros	1997	0.55			56	54	86			3.80	
Costa Rica	2000	2.39	4	3	96	88	108	61	17	4.40	
El Salvador	2002	2.03	6	3	79	87	111	54	17	2.30	13.40
Fiji	1999	2.30	1	1			109	80		5.20	17.00
Gabon	1995	0.29	1			83	129	50		3.90	
Honduras	1997	1.09	1	5	75	70	106		15	4.00	
India	1998	1.13	140	19	57	78	99	49	11	4.10	12.70
Indonesia	2000	0.65	32	9	87	104	110	57	14		
Malaysia	2000	2.39	5	2	89		97	69	26	6.20	26.70
Maldives	2000	2.01		1	97	130	131	55		3.90	11.20
Morocco	2001	1.48	3	2	49	61	101	41	10	5.50	26.10
Nepal	2001	0.31	4	3	42	70	117	40	5	3.70	14.10
Nicaragua	2003	1.78	3	5	67	70	104	54		5.00	13.80
Papua New Guinea	2000	0.58	1	1		60	78	23		2.30	17.50
Paraguay	2000	1.37	1	8	93	89	113	60	16	5.00	11.20

Table A2.2 Global distribution of medical schools and nursing schools (continued)

Country	Year	HRH density	Medical schools	Nursing schools	Adult literacy	Primary school Completion rate (%)	Primary school Enrollment (%)	Secondary school enrollment (%)	Tertiary school enrollment (%)	Public education expenditure Percent of GDP	Public education expenditure Percent of government expenditure
Low-density											
Peru	1999	1.84	17	60	90	99	121			3.30	21.10
São Tomé and Principe	1996	2.04		1		92	125		1		
Solomon Islands	1999	0.98		1						3.60	15.40
Sri Lanka	2000	1.22	6	1	92					3.10	
Suriname	2000	2.07	1	5			127	87			
Thailand	1999	1.92	11	63	93	91	96	83	36	5.40	31.00
Vanuatu	1997	2.46		1		86	111	27		7.30	17.40
Vietnam	2001	1.28	9	4		107	106	67	10		
Cluster cumulative			**301**	**251**							
Cluster weighted average		**1.11**	**88**	**17**	**64**	**83**	**102**	**53**	**13**	**4**	**15**
Moderate-density											
Algeria	1995	3.82	11		67	96	107	68			
Antigua and Barbuda	1999	3.45		1						3.20	
Argentina	1998	3.81	14	25	97	100	120	97	52	4.00	11.80
Barbados	1999	4.92	1	2	100		110	102	38	7.10	18.50
Botswana	1999	2.70		1	77	92	102	73	5	8.60	
Brazil	2001	2.57	82	137	86	79	151	105	16	4.70	12.90
Brunei	2000	4.89		1			109	87	12	4.80	9.10
China	2002	2.68	150	38	91	102	114	68	13	2.10	
Dominica	1997	4.65	1	1		73	100	95		5.10	
Dominican Republic	2000	3.72	10	9	84	80	124	60		2.50	15.70
Ecuador	2000	3.13	8	13	92	99	116	58		1.60	8.00
Egypt, Arab Rep.	2000	4.88	12	11		90	97	85			
Grenada	1997	4.17	1				95	63		4.20	
Guatemala	1999	4.94	2		69	56	102	37		1.70	11.40
Guyana	2000	2.77	1			90				4.10	
Iran, Islamic Rep.	1998	3.51	46		76	105	93	82	20	4.40	20.40
Iraq	2001	3.62	10								
Jamaica	2003	2.50	1		87	84	100	83	16	6.30	11.10
Jordan	2001	4.80	2	7	90	102				5.00	5.00
Kiribati	1998	2.64									
Lebanon	2001	4.43	4	5		71	103	76	42	3.00	11.10
Libya	1997	4.89	4		80		115		48		
Marshall Islands	2000	3.45		1							

A2

QUANTITATIVE INFORMATION

Country	Year	HRH density	Medical schools	Nursing schools	Adult literacy	Primary school		Secondary school enrollment (%)	Tertiary school enrollment (%)	Public education expenditure	
						Completion rate (%)	Enrollment (%)			Percent of GDP	Percent of government expenditure
Moderate-density											
Mauritius	1995	3.18		1	84	105	108	77	11	3.50	12.10
Mexico	2001	3.93	55	4	91	96	110	74	21	4.40	22.60
Micronesia, Fed. Sts.	2000	4.50									
Namibia	1997	3.14			82	92	107	61		8.10	
Oman	2002	4.23	1		72	69	84	77	8	3.90	
Palau	1998	2.56						89	39		
Panama	2000	3.20	2	2	92		109	67		5.90	
Samoa	1999	2.74			99	106	99	74	7	4.20	13.30
Saudi Arabia	2001	4.44	6	4	76	75	68	69	22	9.50	
South Africa	2001	4.57	8	17	85	90	106	85	15	5.50	25.80
St. Vincent and the Grenadines	1997	3.26	2			126	103	69		9.30	
Swaziland	2000	3.38			80	81	102		5	1.50	
Syrian Arab Republic	2001	3.34	3	8	74	89	109	43		4.10	11.10
Tonga	2001	3.70		1		130	112	100	3		
Trinidad and Tobago	1997	3.66	1	3	98	93	101	82	6	4.00	16.70
Tunisia	1997	3.57	4	3	71	91	113	78	21	6.80	17.40
Turkey	2001	4.19	33	10	87		92	73	24	3.50	
Uruguay	2002	4.50	1	3	98	96	109	98	37	2.80	
Venezuela, RB	2001	2.58	9	10	93	55	101	66	23		
Cluster cumulative			**485**	**318**							
Cluster weighted average		**3.05**	**109**	**41**	**89**	**97**	**114**	**74**	**15**	**3**	**17**
High-density											
Albania	2000	5.43	1	4	85	107	107	78	15		
Armenia	2001	8.76	1		98	78	96	86	24	2.90	
Azerbaijan	2001	12.04	1			104	93	80	23	4.20	24.40
Bahamas, The	1998	5.53									
Bahrain	2001	5.72	1		88		98	95		3.00	11.40
Belarus	2001	17.45	4		100		112	85	58	6.00	
Bosnia and Herzegovina	2001	5.73	3		95	81					
Bulgaria	2001	8.26	5		98	96	101	93	40	3.40	
Cuba	2002	13.35	13	24	97	100	102	85	24	8.50	15.10
Estonia	2001	9.78	1	3	100	103	103	110	59	7.50	
Georgia	2002	7.92	2			97	96	73	34		

A2

QUANTITATIVE INFORMATION

Country	Year	HRH density	Medical schools	Nursing schools	Adult literacy	Primary school Completion rate (%)	Primary school Enrollment (%)	Secondary school enrollment (%)	Tertiary school enrollment (%)	Public education expenditure Percent of GDP	Public education expenditure Percent of government expenditure
High-density											
Hungary	2001	11.89	4	9	99		102		40	5.00	14.10
Kazakhstan	2001	9.50	6	1	99	97	97	89	33		
Korea, Dem. Rep.	1995	5.37	10								
Kuwait	2001	5.43	1		82		94	88			
Kyrgyz Republic	2001	10.05	1			93	101	86	41	5.40	
Latvia	2001	8.21	2	2	100	72	99	93	64	5.90	
Lithuania	2001	12.39	2	2	100	103	104	99	59	6.40	
Macedonia, FYR	2001	8.09	1			93	99	85	24		
Moldova	2001	9.21	1		99	81	85	72	28	4.00	15.00
Mongolia	2002	5.95	2	4	98	102	100	71	33	2.30	2.20
Philippines	2002	7.37	28	192	93	105	113	77	31	4.20	20.60
Poland	2000	7.67	14	53		95	100	101	56	5.00	11.40
Qatar	2001	7.15		1			106	89	24	3.60	
Romania	2001	6.20	11	101	98	91	99	82	27	3.50	
Russian Federation	2001	12.51	53		100		109	83	63	4.40	
Seychelles	1996	9.95		1			119	113		7.60	10.70
Slovak Republic	2001	10.63	3	3			103	87	30	4.20	13.80
St. Kitts and Nevis	1997	6.16	2				117	129		2.90	16.40
St. Lucia	1999	7.47		1			113	86		5.80	16.90
Tajikistan	2001	7.20	1		100	100	104	79	14	2.10	11.80
Turkmenistan	1997	10.20	1								
Ukraine	2001	11.16	15		100	95	81	96	53	4.40	15.70
United Arab Emirates	2001	6.21	2	1	76		91	80		1.90	
Uzbekistan	2001	13.67	10	48	99	92					
Cluster cumulative			202	450							
Cluster weighted average		10.12	25	94	98	97	103	86	47	5	17
High-density-low-mortality											
Andorra	2001	5.77									
Australia	2001	10.84	10	45			102	161	63	4.70	
Austria	2001	9.33	3				103	99	57	5.80	12.40
Belgium	2001	15.58	11				105	154	58	5.90	11.60
Canada	2000	12.20	16	31			100	106	59	5.50	
Croatia	2001	7.70	2		98		95	90	34	4.20	10.40
Cyprus	2000	7.84		1	97		97	93	22	5.40	

A2

QUANTITATIVE INFORMATION

Table A2.2 Global distribution of medical schools and nursing schools (continued)

Country	Year	HRH density	Medical schools	Nursing schools	Adult literacy	Primary school Completion rate (%)	Primary school Enrollment (%)	Secondary school enrollment (%)	Tertiary school enrollment (%)	Public education expenditure Percent of GDP	Public education expenditure Percent of government expenditure
High-density-low-mortality											
Czech Republic	2001	13.38	7	5			104	95	30	4.40	9.70
Denmark	2002	13.62	3	22			102		59	8.20	15.30
Finland	2001	25.59	5	3			102	126	85	6.10	12.50
France	2001	10.21	45				105	108	54	5.80	11.50
Germany	2001	13.24	39	44			103	99		4.60	9.70
Greece	2001	7.50	7	3	97		97	96	61	3.80	7.00
Iceland	2001	13.17	1				101	108	48		
Ireland	2001	18.99	5	18					47	4.40	13.20
Israel	2001	10.25	4		95		114	93	53	7.30	
Italy	2001	10.53	31		98		101	96	50	4.50	9.50
Japan	2000	10.41	80	75			101	103	48	3.50	9.30
Korea, Rep.	2000	5.42	48	43			100	94	78	3.80	17.40
Luxembourg	2001	10.45					100	96	10	3.70	8.50
Malta	2001	6.69	1		92		106	90	25	4.90	
Monaco	1995	20.47									
Netherlands	2001	16.73	8	12			108	124	55	4.80	10.70
New Zealand	2001	10.91	2	16			100	112	69	6.10	
Norway	2001	24.89	4	31			102	115	70	6.80	16.20
Portugal	2000	6.98	5	19	92		121	114	50	5.80	13.10
San Marino	1990	7.85									
Singapore	2001	5.64	1	1	93					3.70	23.60
Slovenia	2001	9.36	1	2	100	96	100	106	61		
Spain	2000	6.82	26	57	98		107	114	57	4.50	11.30
Sweden	2000	13.49	6	30			110	149	70	7.80	13.40
Switzerland	2000	12.14	5	43			107	100	42	5.50	15.20
United Kingdom	1993	7.06	27	56			101	158	59	4.50	11.40
United States	2000	13.22	141	523			100	94	71	4.80	
Cluster cumulative			544	1,080							
Cluster weighted average		11.30	69	221	97	96	102	106	61	5	11
Global cumulative			1,631	2,194							
Global minimum		0.12	0	0	16	19	15	6	1	1	2
Global maximum		25.59	150	523	100	130	151	161	85	10	33
Global weighted average		4.04	76	61	78	84	103	70	24	4	14

Table A2.3 Selected health indicators

Country	Year	HRH density	Life expectancy at birth	Under-five mortality rate	Infant mortality rate	Maternal mortality rate	HDI 2000	Poverty level	Female literacy
Low-density-high-mortality									
Afghanistan	2001	0.40	43.0	257[a]	176	820			
Angola	1997	1.27	46.6	260	262	1,300	0.377		
Benin	1995	0.34	53.0	158	132	880	0.411		25
Burkina Faso	2001	0.34	44.2	197	167	1,400	0.330	61.2	15
Burundi	2000	0.34	42.0	190	142	1,900	0.337	58.4	42
Cambodia	2000	1.00	53.8	138	137	590	0.556		58
Cameroon	1996	0.45	50.1	155	103	720	0.499	33.4	65
Central African Republic	1995	0.17	43.4	180	160	1,200	0.363	66.6	37
Chad	2001	0.20	48.4	200	163	1,500	0.376	2.0	36
Congo, Dem. Rep.	1996	0.51	45.6	205	176	940	0.363		52
Congo, Rep.	1995	2.35	51.3	108	92	1,100	0.502		76
Côte d'Ivoire	1996	0.55	45.8	175	141	1,200	0.396	12.3	38
Djibouti	1999	0.79	46.3	143	138	520	0.462		56
Equatorial Guinea	1996	0.67	51.0	153	125	1,400	0.664		76
Eritrea	1996	0.21	51.0	111	85	1,100	0.446		46
Ethiopia	2002	0.23	42.3	172	143	1,800	0.359	81.9	32
Gambia, The	1997	0.25	53.3	126	92	1,100	0.463	59.3	31
Ghana	2002	0.93	57.0	100	70	590	0.567	44.8	65
Guinea	2000	0.56	46.3	169	153	1,200	0.425		
Guinea-Bissau	1996	1.39	44.9	211	177	910	0.373		25
Haiti	1998	0.36	52.7	123	89	1,100	0.467		49
Kenya	1995	1.03	47.0	122	90	1,300	0.489	23.0	77
Lao PDR	1996	1.62	53.7	100	106	650	0.525	26.3	54
Lesotho	1995	1.12	41.4	132	98	530	0.510	43.1	94
Liberia	1997	0.12	47.2	235[a]	231	1,000			
Madagascar	2001	0.36	54.7	136	131	580	0.468	49.1	61
Malawi	2003	0.31	38.8	183	199	580	0.387	41.7	48
Mali	2000	0.19	42.0	231	205	630	0.337	72.8	17
Mauritania	1995	0.86	50.8	183	148	870	0.454	28.6	31
Mozambique	2000	0.31	42.4	197	149	980	0.356	37.9	30
Myanmar	2000	0.78	56.7	109	112	170	0.549		81
Niger	2002	0.30	45.4	265	239	920	0.292	61.4	9
Nigeria	2000	1.45	46.8	183	134	1,100	0.463	70.2	58
Pakistan	2001	1.13	63.0	109	84	200	0.499	13.4	29
Rwanda	2002	0.23	39.9	183	152	2,300	0.422	35.7	62
Senegal	1995	0.36	52.3	138	104	1,200	0.430	26.3	29
Sierra Leone	1996	0.45	37.3	316	258	2,100	0.275	57.0	
Somalia	1997	0.23	47.2	225[a]	157	1,600			
Sudan	2000	1.01	57.5	107	107	1,500	0.503		48
Tanzania	2002	0.39	44.4	165	123	1,100	0.400	19.9	68

Table A2.3 Selected health indicators (continued)

Country	Year	HRH density	Life expectancy at birth	Under-five mortality rate	Infant mortality rate	Maternal mortality rate	HDI 2000	Poverty level	Female literacy
Low-density-high-mortality									
Togo	2001	0.30	49.3	141	105	980	0.501		44
Uganda	2002	0.14	42.5	124	120	1,100	0.489	82.2	58
Yemen, Rep.	2001	0.67	56.5	107	97	850	0.470	15.7	27
Zambia	1995	1.20	38.0	202	168	870	0.386	63.7	73
Zimbabwe	2002	0.60	39.9	123	98	610	0.496	36.0	86
Cluster weighted average		**0.77**	**50.1**	**157**	**128**	**920**		**44**	**48**
Low-density									
Bangladesh	2001	0.47	61.2	77	77	600	0.502	36.0	31
Belize	2000	2.31	73.9	40	23	140	0.776		93
Bhutan	1999	0.28	62.2	95	68	500	0.511		
Bolivia	2001	1.05	62.6	77	66	550	0.672	14.4	80
Cape Verde	1996	0.73	68.8	38	35	190	0.727		67
Chile	2003	1.72	75.9	12	9	33	0.831		96
Colombia	2002	1.90	71.4	23	20	120	0.779	14.4	92
Comoros	1997	0.55	60.7	79	75	570	0.528		49
Costa Rica	2000	2.39	77.5	11	10	35	0.832	6.9	96
El Salvador	2002	2.03	69.8	39	28	180	0.719	21.4	77
Fiji	1999	2.30	69.1	21	24	20	0.754		91
Gabon	1995	0.29	52.7	90	74	620	0.653		
Honduras	1997	1.09	66.0	38	35	220	0.667	23.8	76
India	1998	1.13	62.9	93	76	440	0.590	34.7	46
Indonesia	2000	0.65	66.0	45	40	470	0.682	7.2	83
Malaysia	2000	2.39	72.5	8	7	39	0.790	2.0	84
Maldives	2000	2.01	68.3	77	38	390	0.751		97
Morocco	2001	1.48	67.7	44	56	390	0.606	2.0	37
Nepal	2001	0.31	58.9	91	86	830	0.499	37.7	25
Nicaragua	2003	1.78	68.5	43	35	250	0.643	82.3	67
Papua New Guinea	2000	0.58	57.2	94	74	390	0.548		58
Paraguay	2000	1.37	70.4	30	27	170	0.751	19.5	93
Peru	1999	1.84	69.3	39	37	240	0.752	15.5	86
São Tomé and Príncipe	1996	2.04	65.1	74	107		0.639		
Solomon Islands	1999	0.98	68.6	24	66	60	0.632		
Sri Lanka	2000	1.22	73.0	19	15	60	0.730	6.6	89
Suriname	2000	2.07	70.2	32	25	230	0.762		
Thailand	1999	1.92	68.8	28	36	44	0.768	2.0	94
Vanuatu	1997	2.46	68.1	42	50		0.568		
Vietnam	2001	1.28	69.1	38	28	95	0.688	17.7	91
Cluster weighted average		**1.11**	**64.5**	**74**	**63**	**403**		**27**	**57**

A2

QUANTITATIVE INFORMATION

Table A2.3 Selected health indicators (continued)

Country	Year	HRH density	Life expectancy at birth	Under-five mortality rate	Infant mortality rate	Maternal mortality rate	HDI 2000	Poverty level	Female literacy
Moderate-density									
Algeria	1995	3.82	70.5	49	36	150	0.704	2.0	58
Antigua and Barbuda	1999	3.45	75.1	14	18		0.798		
Argentina	1998	3.81	73.9	19	18	84	0.849		97
Barbados	1999	4.92	75.4	14	19	33	0.888		100
Botswana	1999	2.70	39.0	110	59	480	0.614	23.5	81
Brazil	2001	2.57	68.1	36	38	260	0.777	9.9	87
Brunei	2000	4.89	76.3	6	10	22	0.872		88
China	2002	2.68	70.3	39	38	60	0.721	16.1	79
Dominica	1997	4.65	76.3	15	12		0.776		
Dominican Republic	2000	3.72	67.3	47	41	110	0.737	2.0	84
Ecuador	2000	3.13	69.7	30	27	210	0.731	20.2	90
Egypt, Arab Rep.	2000	4.88	67.8	41	38	170	0.648	3.1	45
Grenada	1997	4.17	72.5	25	18		0.738		
Guatemala	1999	4.94	65.0	58	39	270	0.652	16.0	62
Guyana	2000	2.77	62.9	72	45	150	0.740	2.0	98
Iran, Islamic Rep.	1998	3.51	68.8	42	37	130	0.719	2.0	70
Iraq	2001	3.62	61.1	125[a]	103	370			
Jamaica	2003	2.50	75.3	20	12	120	0.757	2.0	91
Jordan	2001	4.80	71.5	33	17	41	0.743	2.0	85
Kiribati	1998	2.64	61.9	70[a]	61				
Lebanon	2001	4.43	70.4	32	22	130	0.752		81
Libya	1997	4.89	71.5	19	25	120	0.783		69
Marshall Islands	2000	3.45	65.2	68[a]	26				
Mauritius	1995	3.18	71.7	19	13	45	0.779		82
Mexico	2001	3.93	73.1	29	25	67	0.800	8.0	90
Micronesia, Fed. Sts.	2000	4.50	68.0	24[a]	50				
Namibia	1997	3.14	47.2	67	69	370	0.627	34.9	82
Oman	2002	4.23	73.6	13	19	120	0.755		64
Palau	1998	2.56	70.4	29[a]	18				
Panama	2000	3.20	74.6	25	19	100	0.788	7.6	91
Samoa	1999	2.74	69.1	25	16	15	0.775		98
Saudi Arabia	2001	4.44	72.5	28	24	23	0.769		68
South Africa	2001	4.57	47.8	71	73	340	0.684	2.0	85
St. Vincent and the Grenadines	1997	3.26	72.9	25	17		0.755		
Swaziland	2000	3.38	45.4	149	80	370	0.547		79
Syrian Arab Republic	2001	3.34	69.7	28	24	200	0.685		62
Tonga	2001	3.70	71.0	21[a]	19				
Trinidad and Tobago	1997	3.66	72.6	20	18	65	0.802	12.4	98
Tunisia	1997	3.57	72.1	27	22	70	0.740	2.0	62
Turkey	2001	4.19	69.6	43	34	55	0.734	2.0	77

Table A2.3 Selected health indicators (continued)

Country	Year	HRH density	Life expectancy at birth	Under-five mortality rate	Infant mortality rate	Maternal mortality rate	HDI 2000	Poverty level	Female literacy
Moderate-density									
Uruguay	2002	4.50	74.4	16	14	50	0.834	2.0	98
Venezuela, RB	2001	2.58	73.4	22	20	43	0.775	15.0	92
Cluster weighted average		**3.05**	**69.5**	**40**	**37**	**99**		**13**	**79**
High-density									
Albania	2000	5.43	74.0	30	26	31	0.735		78
Armenia	2001	8.76	73.6	35	28	29	0.729	12.8	98
Azerbaijan	2001	12.04	65.2	105	78	37	0.744	3.7	
Bahamas, The	1998	5.53	69.4	16	8	10	0.812		96
Bahrain	2001	5.72	73.1	16	6	38	0.839		83
Belarus	2001	17.45	68.0	20	9	33	0.804	2.0	100
Bosnia and Herzegovina	2001	5.73	73.3	18	17	15	0.777		
Bulgaria	2001	8.26	71.5	16	11	23	0.795	4.7	98
Cuba	2002	13.35	76.5	9	8	24	0.806		97
Estonia	2001	9.78	70.6	12	9	80	0.833	2.0	100
Georgia	2002	7.92	73.0	29	24	22	0.746	2.0	
Hungary	2001	11.89	71.2	9	8	23	0.837	2.0	99
Kazakhstan	2001	9.50	64.2	76	41	80	0.765	1.5	99
Korea, Dem. Rep.	1995	5.37	61.1	55[a]	33	35			
Kuwait	2001	5.43	76.6	10	8	25	0.820		80
Kyrgyz Republic	2001	10.05	66.4	61	54	80	0.727	2.0	
Latvia	2001	8.21	70.4	21	9	70	0.811	2.0	100
Lithuania	2001	12.39	72.6	9	8	27	0.824	2.0	100
Macedonia, FYR	2001	8.09	72.8	26	12	17	0.784	2.0	
Moldova	2001	9.21	67.5	32	17	63	0.700	22.0	98
Mongolia	2002	5.95	65.1	76	57	65	0.661	13.9	98
Philippines	2002	7.37	69.3	38	29	240	0.751	14.6	95
Poland	2000	7.67	73.3	9	7	12	0.841	2.0	100
Qatar	2001	7.15	74.7	16	13	41	0.826		84
Romania	2001	6.20	69.9	21	26	62	0.773	2.1	97
Russian Federation	2001	12.51	65.3	21	16	74	0.779	6.1	99
Seychelles	1996	9.95	72.3	17	11		0.840		
Slovak Republic	2001	10.63	73.1	9	8	14	0.836	2.0	
St. Kitts and Nevis	1997	6.16	70.8	24	15		0.808		
St. Lucia	1999	7.47	71.8	19	14		0.775		
Tajikistan	2001	7.20	67.3	72	75	120	0.677	10.3	99
Turkmenistan	1997	10.20	65.1	99	52	65	0.748	12.1	
Ukraine	2001	11.16	68.2	20	10	45	0.766	2.9	100
United Arab Emirates	2001	6.21	75.3	9	9	30	0.816		80
Uzbekistan	2001	13.67	67.9	68	42	60	0.729	19.1	99
Cluster weighted average		**10.12**	**68.1**	**31**	**22**	**82**		**7**	**98**

Country	Year	HRH density	Life expectancy at birth	Under-five mortality rate	Infant mortality rate	Maternal mortality rate	HDI 2000	Poverty level	Female literacy
High-density-low mortality									
Andorra	2001	5.77		7[a]	5				
Australia	2001	10.84	78.9	6	5	6	0.939		
Austria	2001	9.33	78.2	5	4	11	0.929		
Belgium	2001	15.58	78.2	6	5	33	0.937		
Canada	2000	12.20	78.9	7	5	6	0.937		
Croatia	2001	7.70	73.3	8	8	18	0.818	2.0	97
Cyprus	2000	7.84	77.9	6	6		0.891		96
Czech Republic	2001	13.38	74.8	5	3	14	0.861	2.0	
Denmark	2002	13.62	76.5	4	5	15	0.930		
Finland	2001	25.59	77.5	5	3	6	0.930		
France	2001	10.21	78.9	6	5	20	0.925		
Germany	2001	13.24	77.7	5	5	12	0.921		
Greece	2001	7.50	77.9	5	6	2	0.892		96
Iceland	2001	13.17	79.5	4	2	16	0.942		
Ireland	2001	18.99	76.3	6	6	9	0.930		
Israel	2001	10.25	78.4	6	6	8	0.905		93
Italy	2001	10.53	78.7	6	5	11	0.916		98
Japan	2000	10.41	81.1	5	3	12	0.932		
Korea, Rep.	2000	5.42	73.3	5	6	20	0.879	2.0	97
Luxembourg	2001	10.45	77.3	5	3		0.930		
Malta	2001	6.69	78.0	5	6		0.856		93
Monaco	1995	20.47		5[a]	5				
Netherlands	2001	16.73	78.0	6	5	10	0.938		
New Zealand	2001	10.91	78.2	6	5	15	0.917		
Norway	2001	24.89	78.6	4	4	9	0.944		
Portugal	2000	6.98	75.6	6	6	12	0.896	2.0	90
San Marino	1990	7.85		6[a]	6				
Singapore	2001	5.64	78.0	4	3	9	0.884		89
Slovenia	2001	9.36	75.3	5	4	17	0.881	2.0	100
Spain	2000	6.82	78.2	6	4	8	0.918		97
Sweden	2000	13.49	79.6	3	2	8	0.941		
Switzerland	2000	12.14	79.9	6	4	8	0.932		
United Kingdom	1993	7.06	77.3	7	6	10	0.930		
United States	2000	13.22	77.0	8	8	12	0.937		
Cluster weighted average		**11.30**	**77.9**	**6**	**5**	**12**		**2**	**97**
Global minimum		**0.12**	**37.3**	**3**	**2**	**2**		**2**	**9**
Global maximum		**25.59**	**81.1**	**316**	**262**	**2,300**		**52**	**100**
Global weighted average		**4.04**	**66.5**	**60**	**51**	**286**		**21**	**69**

a. Data are for the year 2000 from the World Bank's *World Development Indicators 2004*.

Table A2.4 Health workforce financing

Country	Year	HRH density	GNI PPP per capita	Total health spending per capita		External resources for health per capita		External resources for HRH per capita	
				US dollars	PPP	US dollars	Share of total health spending (%)	Minimum (US dollars)	Maximum (US dollars)
Low-density-high-mortality									
Afghanistan	2001	0.40		8	34	0.90	11.2	0.27	0.45
Angola	1997	1.27	1,690	31	70	4.40	14.2	1.32	2.20
Benin	1995	0.34	970	16	39	3.44	21.5	1.03	1.72
Burkina Faso	2001	0.34	1,120	6	27	1.54	25.6	0.46	0.77
Burundi	2000	0.34	680	4	19	1.75	43.7	0.52	0.87
Cambodia	2000	1.00	1,790	30	184	5.91	19.7	1.77	2.96
Cameroon	1996	0.45	1,580	20	42	1.26	6.3	0.38	0.63
Central African Republic	1995	0.17	1,300	12	58	3.89	32.4	1.17	1.94
Chad	2001	0.20	1,060	5	17	3.15	62.9	0.94	1.57
Congo, Dem. Rep.	1996	0.51	680	5	12	0.90	18.0	0.27	0.45
Congo, Rep.	1995	2.35	630	18	22	0.59	3.3	0.18	0.30
Côte d'Ivoire	1996	0.55	1,400	41	127	1.31	3.2	0.39	0.66
Djibouti	1999	0.79	2,420	58	90	17.40	30.0	5.22	8.70
Equatorial Guinea	1996	0.67		76	106	8.06	10.6	2.42	4.03
Eritrea	1996	0.21	1,030	10	36	5.23	52.3	1.57	2.62
Ethiopia	2002	0.23	800	3	14	1.03	34.3	0.31	0.51
Gambia, The	1997	0.25	2,010	19	78	5.05	26.6	1.52	2.53
Ghana	2002	0.93	2,170	12	60	2.78	23.2	0.84	1.39
Guinea	2000	0.56	1,900	13	61	2.67	20.5	0.80	1.33
Guinea-Bissau	1996	1.39	890	8	37	3.09	38.6	0.93	1.54
Haiti	1998	0.36	1,870	22	56	9.44	42.9	2.83	4.72
Kenya	1995	1.03	970	29	114	2.84	9.8	0.85	1.42
Lao PDR	1996	1.62	1,540	10	51	2.11	21.1	0.63	1.06
Lesotho	1995	1.12	2,980	23	101	1.38	6.0	0.41	0.69
Liberia	1997	0.12		1	127	0.57	57.2	0.17	0.29
Madagascar	2001	0.36	820	6	20	2.21	36.8	0.66	1.10
Malawi	2003	0.31	560	13	39	3.45	26.5	1.03	1.72
Mali	2000	0.19	770	11	30	2.29	20.8	0.69	1.14
Mauritania	1995	0.86	1,940	12	45	2.78	23.2	0.84	1.39
Mozambique	2000	0.31	1,050	11	47	4.06	36.9	1.22	2.03
Myanmar	2000	0.78		197	26	0.39	0.2	0.12	0.20
Niger	2002	0.30	880	6	22	1.01	16.9	0.30	0.51
Nigeria	2000	1.45	790	15	31	1.07	7.1	0.32	0.53
Pakistan	2001	1.13	1,860	16	85	0.30	1.9	0.09	0.15
Rwanda	2002	0.23	1,240	11	44	2.72	24.7	0.82	1.36
Senegal	1995	0.36	1,480	22	63	4.44	20.2	1.33	2.22
Sierra Leone	1996	0.45	460	7	26	1.76	25.1	0.53	0.88

Table A2.4 *Health workforce financing (continued)*

Country	Year	HRH density	GNI PPP per capita	Total health spending per capita		External resources for health per capita		External resources for HRH per capita	
				US dollars	PPP	US dollars	Share of total health spending (%)	Minimum (US dollars)	Maximum (US dollars)
Low-density-high-mortality									
Somalia	1997	0.23		6		0.56	9.3	0.17	0.28
Sudan	2000	1.01	1,750	14	39	0.38	2.7	0.11	0.19
Tanzania	2002	0.39	520	12	26	3.54	29.5	1.06	1.77
Togo	2001	0.30	1,620	8	45	0.65	8.1	0.19	0.32
Uganda	2002	0.14	1,460	14	57	3.47	24.8	1.04	1.74
Yemen, Rep.	2001	0.67	730	20	69	0.74	3.7	0.22	0.37
Zambia	1995	1.20	750	19	52	9.25	48.7	2.78	4.63
Zimbabwe	2002	0.60	2,220	45	142	3.51	7.8	1.05	1.76
Cluster weighted average		**0.77**	**1,224**	**25**	**51**	**1.75**	**15.51**	**0.53**	**0.88**
Low-density									
Bangladesh	2001	0.47	1,600	12	58	1.60	13.3	0.48	0.80
Belize	2000	2.31	5,150	167	278	10.19	6.1	3.06	5.09
Bhutan	1999	0.28		9	64	3.44	38.2	1.03	1.72
Bolivia	2001	1.05	2,240	49	125	5.98	12.2	1.79	2.99
Cape Verde	1996	0.73	5,540	46	134	9.34	20.3	2.80	4.67
Chile	2003	1.72	8,840	303	792	0.30	0.1	0.09	0.15
Colombia	2002	1.90	6,790	105	356	0.21	0.2	0.06	0.11
Comoros	1997	0.55	1,890	9	29	3.59	39.9	1.08	1.80
Costa Rica	2000	2.39	9,260	293	562	3.81	1.3	1.14	1.90
El Salvador	2002	2.03	5,160	174	376	1.57	0.9	0.47	0.78
Fiji	1999	2.30	4,920	79	224	7.98	10.1	2.39	3.99
Gabon	1995	0.29	5,190	127	197	2.29	1.8	0.69	1.14
Honduras	1997	1.09	2,760	59	153	4.43	7.5	1.33	2.21
India	1998	1.13	2,820	24	80	0.01	0.4	0.03	0.05
Indonesia	2000	0.65	2,830	16	77	1.04	6.5	0.31	0.52
Malaysia	2000	2.39	7,910	143	345	—	—	—	—
Maldives	2000	2.01		98	263	1.86	1.9	0.56	0.93
Morocco	2001	1.48	3,500	59	199	0.83	1.4	0.25	0.41
Nepal	2001	0.31	1,360	12	63	1.13	9.4	0.34	0.56
Nicaragua	2003	1.78		60	158	4.62	7.7	1.39	2.31
Papua New Guinea	2000	0.58	2,450	24	144	5.09	21.2	1.53	2.54
Paraguay	2000	1.37	5,180	97	332	1.94	2.0	0.58	0.97
Peru	1999	1.84	4,470	97	231	1.65	1.7	0.49	0.82
São Tomé and Principe	1996	2.04		7	22	3.95	56.4	1.18	1.97
Solomon Islands	1999	0.98	1,910	40	133	6.36	15.9	1.91	3.18
Sri Lanka	2000	1.22	3,260	30	122	0.93	3.1	0.28	0.47
Suriname	2000	2.07		153	398	18.97	12.4	5.69	9.49

Country	Year	HRH density	GNI PPP per capita	Total health spending per capita		External resources for health per capita		External resources for HRH per capita	
				US dollars	PPP	US dollars	Share of total health spending (%)	Minimum (US dollars)	Maximum (US dollars)
Low-density									
Thailand	1999	1.92	6,230	69	254	0.07	0.1	0.02	0.03
Vanuatu	1997	2.46	3,110	42	107	3.53	8.4	1.06	1.76
Vietnam	2001	1.28	2,070	21	134	0.55	2.6	0.16	0.27
Cluster weighted average		**1.11**	**3,084**	**33**	**113**	**0.54**	**2.76**	**0.16**	**0.27**
Moderate-density									
Algeria	1995	3.82	5,910	73	169	0.07	0.1	0.02	0.04
Antigua and Barbuda	1999	3.45	9,550	531	614	15.40	2.9	4.62	7.70
Argentina	1998	3.81	10,980	679	1130	2.04	0.3	0.61	1.02
Barbados	1999	4.92	15,110	613	940	28.20	4.6	8.46	14.01
Botswana	1999	2.70	7,410	190	381	0.76	0.4	0.23	0.38
Brazil	2001	2.57	7,070	222	573	1.11	0.5	0.33	0.56
Brunei	2000	4.89		453	638				
China	2002	2.68	3,950	49	224	0.01	0.2	0.03	0.05
Dominica	1997	4.65	4,920	203	312	1.83	0.9	0.55	0.91
Dominican Republic	2000	3.72	6,650	153	353	2.75	1.8	0.83	1.38
Ecuador	2000	3.13	2,960	76	177	1.44	1.9	0.43	0.72
Egypt, Arab Rep.	2000	4.88	3,560	46	153	0.92	2.0	0.28	0.46
Grenada	1997	4.17	6,290	262	445	—	—	—	—
Guatemala	1999	4.94	4,380	86	199	1.20	1.4	0.36	0.60
Guyana	2000	2.77	4,280	50	215	1.10	2.2	0.33	0.55
Iran, Islamic Rep.	1998	3.51	5,940	350	422	0.35	0.1	0.11	0.18
Iraq	2001	3.62		225	97	0.23	0.1	0.07	0.11
Jamaica	2003	2.50	3,490	191	253	5.73	3.0	1.72	2.87
Jordan	2001	4.80	3,880	163	412	7.17	4.4	2.15	3.59
Kiribati	1998	2.64		40	143	1.76	4.4	0.53	0.88
Lebanon	2001	4.43	4,400	500	673	1.00	0.2	0.30	0.50
Libya	1997	4.89		143	239	—	—	—	—
Marshall Islands	2000	3.45		190	343	48.26	25.4	14.48	24.13
Mauritius	1995	3.18	9,860	128	323	2.05	1.6	0.61	1.02
Mexico	2001	3.93	8,240	370	544	1.85	0.5	0.56	0.93
Micronesia, Fed. Sts.	2000	4.50		172	319	27.86	16.2	8.36	13.93
Namibia	1997	3.14	7,410	110	330	4.29	3.9	1.29	2.15
Oman	2002	4.23	10,720	225	343	—	—	—	—
Palau	1998	2.56		426	886	50.27	11.8	15.08	25.13
Panama	2000	3.20	5,440	258	458	1.55	0.6	0.46	0.77
Samoa	1999	2.74	6,130	74	199	11.54	15.6	3.46	5.77
Saudi Arabia	2001	4.44	13,290	375	591	—	—	—	—

Table A2.4 Health workforce financing (continued)

Country	Year	HRH density	GNI PPP per capita	Total health spending per capita		External resources for health per capita		External resources for HRH per capita	
				US dollars	PPP	US dollars	Share of total health spending (%)	Minimum (US dollars)	Maximum (US dollars)
Moderate-density									
South Africa	2001	4.57	10,910	222	652	0.89	0.4	0.27	0.44
St. Vincent and the Grenadines	1997	3.26		178	358	0.53	0.3	0.16	0.27
Swaziland	2000	3.38	4,430	41	167	3.24	7.9	0.97	1.62
Syrian Arab Republic	2001	3.34	3,160	41	266	0.21	0.5	0.06	0.10
Tonga	2001	3.70		73	223	15.11	20.7	4.53	7.56
Trinidad and Tobago	1997	3.66	8,620	279	388	10.60	3.8	3.18	5.30
Tunisia	1997	3.57	6,090	134	463	0.80	0.6	0.24	0.40
Turkey	2001	4.19	5,830	109	294	—	—	—	—
Uruguay	2002	4.50	8,250	603	971	4.82	0.8	1.45	2.41
Venezuela, RB	2001	2.58	5,590	307	386	0.31	0.1	0.09	0.15
Cluster weighted average		**3.05**	**5,027**	**120**	**310**	**0.45**	**0.35**	**0.13**	**0.22**
High-density									
Albania	2000	5.43	3,810	48	150	1.63	3.4	0.49	0.82
Armenia	2001	8.76	2,730	54	273	2.00	3.7	0.60	1.00
Azerbaijan	2001	12.04	2,890	11	48	0.85	7.7	0.25	0.42
Bahamas, The	1998	5.53	15,680	864	1220	2.59	0.3	0.78	1.30
Bahrain	2001	5.72	15,390	500	664	—	—	—	—
Belarus	2001	17.45	7,630	68	464	—	—	—	—
Bosnia and Herzegovina	2001	5.73	6,250	85	268	2.04	2.4	0.61	1.02
Bulgaria	2001	8.26	6,740	81	303	1.70	2.1	0.51	0.85
Cuba	2002	13.35		185	229	0.37	0.2	0.11	0.19
Estonia	2001	9.78	9,650	226	562	—	—	—	—
Georgia	2002	7.92	2,580	22	108	1.12	5.1	0.34	0.56
Hungary	2001	11.89	11,990	345	914	—	—	—	—
Kazakhstan	2001	9.50	6,150	44	204	1.54	3.5	0.46	0.77
Korea, Dem. Rep.	1995	5.37		22	44	0.07	0.3	0.02	0.03
Kuwait	2001	5.43	21,530	537	612	—	—	—	—
Kyrgyz Republic	2001	10.05	2,630	12	108				
Latvia	2001	8.21	7,760	210	509	1.47	0.7	0.44	0.74
Lithuania	2001	12.39	8,350	206	478	2.06	1.0	0.62	1.03
Macedonia, FYR	2001	8.09	6,040	115	331	4.03	3.5	1.21	2.01
Moldova	2001	9.21	2,300	18	100	1.53	8.5	0.46	0.77
Mongolia	2002	5.95	1,710	25	122	3.85	15.4	1.16	1.93
Philippines	2002	7.37	4,070	30	169	1.05	3.5	0.32	0.53
Poland	2000	7.67	9,370	289	629	—	—	—	—
Qatar	2001	7.15		885	782	—	—	—	—
Romania	2001	6.20	5,780	117	460	1.17	1.0	0.35	0.59

Country	Year	HRH density	GNI PPP per capita	Total health spending per capita		External resources for health per capita		External resources for HRH per capita	
				US dollars	PPP	US dollars	Share of total health spending (%)	Minimum (US dollars)	Maximum (US dollars)
High-density									
Russian Federation	2001	12.51	6,880	115	454	3.57	3.1	1.07	1.78
Seychelles	1996	9.95		450	770	53.55	11.9	16.07	26.78
Slovak Republic	2001	10.63	11,780	216	681	—	—	—	—
St. Kitts and Nevis	1997	6.16		393	576	22.01	5.6	6.60	11.00
St. Lucia	1999	7.47		199	272	1.19	0.6	0.36	0.60
Tajikistan	2001	7.20	1,140	6	43	0.35	5.9	0.11	0.18
Turkmenistan	1997	10.20	4,240	57	245	0.34	0.6	0.10	0.17
Ukraine	2001	11.16	4,270	33	176	0.23	0.7	0.07	0.12
United Arab Emirates	2001	6.21		849	921	—	—	—	—
Uzbekistan	2001	13.67	2,410	17	91	0.29	1.7	0.09	0.14
Cluster weighted average		**10.12**	**5,921**	**104**	**332**	**1.53**	**2.32**	**0.46**	**0.77**
High-density-low-mortality									
Andorra	2001	5.77		1233	1821	—	—	—	—
Australia	2001	10.84	24,630	1741	2532	—	—	—	—
Austria	2001	9.33	26,380	1866	2259	—	—	—	—
Belgium	2001	15.58	26,150	1983	2481	—	—	—	—
Canada	2000	12.20	26,530	2163	2792	—	—	—	—
Croatia	2001	7.70	8,930	394	726	0.39	0.1	0.12	0.20
Cyprus	2000	7.84	21,110	932	941	21.44	2.3	6.43	10.72
Czech Republic	2001	13.38	14,320	407	1129	—	—	—	—
Denmark	2002	13.62	28,490	2545	2503	—	—	—	—
Finland	2001	25.59	24,030	1631	1845	—	—	—	—
France	2001	10.21	24,080	2109	2567	—	—	—	—
Germany	2001	13.24	25,240	2412	2820	—	—	—	—
Greece	2001	7.50	17,520	1001	1522	—	—	—	—
Iceland	2001	13.17	28,850	2441	2643	—	—	—	—
Ireland	2001	18.99	27,170	1714	1935	—	—	—	—
Israel	2001	10.25	19,630	1641	1839	1.64	0.1	0.49	0.82
Italy	2001	10.53	24,530	1584	2204	—	—	—	—
Japan	2000	10.41	25,550	2627	2131	—	—	—	—
Korea, Rep.	2000	5.42	15,060	532	948	—	—	—	—
Luxembourg	2001	10.45	48,560	2600	2905	—	—	—	—
Malta	2001	6.69	13,140	808	813	—	—	—	—
Monaco	1995	20.47		1653	2016	—	—	—	—
Netherlands	2001	16.73	27,390	2138	2612	—	—	—	—
New Zealand	2001	10.91	18,250	1073	1724	—	—	—	—
Norway	2001	24.89	29,340	2981	2920	—	—	—	—

Country	Year	HRH density	GNI PPP per capita	Total health spending per capita		External resources for health per capita		External resources for HRH per capita	
				US dollars	PPP	US dollars	Share of total health spending (%)	Minimum (US dollars)	Maximum (US dollars)
High-density-low-mortality									
Portugal	2000	6.98	17,710	982	1618	—	—	—	—
San Marino	1990	7.85		1222	1711	—	—	—	—
Singapore	2001	5.64	22,850	816	993	—	—	—	—
Slovenia	2001	9.36	17,060	821	1545	—	—	—	—
Spain	2000	6.82	19,860	1088	1607	—	—	—	—
Sweden	2000	13.49	23,800	2150	2270	—	—	—	—
Switzerland	2000	12.14	30,970	3774	3322	—	—	—	—
United Kingdom	1993	7.06	24,340	1835	1989	—	—	—	—
United States	2000	13.22	34,280	4887	4887	—	—	—	—
Cluster weighted average		**11.30**	**26,828**	**2,822**	**2,994**	**0.03**	**0.00**	**0.01**	**0.02**
Global minimum		**0.12**	**460.00**	**1.00**	**12.00**	**—**	**—**	**—**	**—**
Global maximum		**25.59**	**48,560.00**	**4,887.00**	**4,887.00**	**53.55**	**62.90**	**16.07**	**26.78**
Global weighted average		**4.04**	**7,485**	**497**	**634**	**0.68**	**3.29**	**0.20**	**0.34**

Joint Learning Initiative

The Joint Learning Initiative on Human Resources for Health and Development (JLI) was launched in November 2002 in recognition of the centrality of the workforce for global health. At that time, human resources for health was neglected as a critical resource for the performance of health systems. Put simply, the workforce was invisible in the policy agenda. Political deliberations and social advocacy had appropriately focused on increasing financing and lowering prices of antiretroviral drugs for saving lives at risk to HIV/AIDS. To the founders of the JLI, it became progressively clear that the workforce, the human backbone of all health action, was comparatively overlooked. Human resources presented both a huge opportunity as well as a major bottleneck to overcoming global health challenges.

The JLI was crafted as a multistakeholder participatory learning process with the dual aims of landscaping human resources and recommending strategies for strengthening the workforce for health systems.

The information that follows describes the JLI goals; working group co-chairs and members; reports and working papers; consultations, workshops, and activities. Also appended are the JLI secretariat, the research and writing team, and acknowledgment of financial partners.

JLI was designed as an open, collaborative, and consultative process involving a diverse membership from around the world. More than 100 members joined seven working groups to pursue—in a decentralized manner—a learning agenda crafted by the working groups. Each of the seven working groups was assigned a theme— history, supply, demand, Africa, priority diseases, innovation, and coordination—and encouraged to pursue that theme. This open, unstructured design was intended to encourage creativity, innovation, and an unimpeded dialogue enabling JLI to bring out the best of the combined expertise of its diverse participants. Over the two years of its life, the JLI has not only conducted research and analysis but also consulted widely. Its learnings—crystallized in its papers, reports, and especially the JLI Strategy Report—are intended to help accelerate community, country, and global strategies to strengthen the health workforce in all countries, but especially those facing health crises.

JLI's work was conducted in three phases. A preparatory phase from spring 2001 to fall 2002 developed a conceptual framework, engaged key partners, and established leadership of the seven working groups.

A second phase over calendar year 2003 was marked by working group activities, the review of existing literature, and the commissioning of new research and analyses—all aimed at generating fresh insights on human resources for health. A major effort was made to extend outreach through more than 30 workshops and meetings. These consultations were conducted in all parts of the world, usually in collaboration with hosts and partners, and they expanded the interactive space of JLI participants. Consultations included not only papers and professional dialogue but also direct conversation with health workers, listening to the voices of the workers themselves.

The third phase beginning in January 2004 was launched by a successful JLI presentation in Geneva at the High Level Forum for the Health MDGs sponsored by the WHO and the World Bank. JLI advocacy was accelerated as its research and learnings were increasingly culled for quality and consolidated for policy-oriented recommendations. To emphasize the importance of country strategies, JLI engaged in a half dozen interactive country consultations—South Africa, Kenya, Brazil, Thailand, and Lithuania. The learnings from these country-based exchanges were integrated into the JLI Strategy Report.

As a unique endeavor, the JLI process was supported by three secretariat bases—in New York City at the Rockefeller Foundation and in Boston at John Snow Inc., and the Global Equity Initiative of Harvard University. Access to JLI research is available on the website: www.globalhealthtrust.org. This JLI Strategy Report represented a true team effort, with all working groups contributing data, analyses, and recommendations. Specific contributions of researchers and writers are listed. Based at the secretariat of the Global Equity Initiative, the JLI Strategy Report research, writing, and production was directed by Lincoln Chen backed by the research coordination of Sarah Michael and Piya Hanvoravongchai.

JLI thanks and acknowledges the funding partners who offered flexible financing for participation and learning. We thank in particular the Rockefeller Foundation, which launched the JLI, Swedish Sida, which provided unrestricted support at a critical juncture, the Bill & Melinda Gates Foundation, which encouraged openness to learning, and The Atlantic Philanthropies, which provided exceptional support for our South African and overall work. Other participating contributors were the Open Society Institute (OSI), Canadian International Development Agency (CIDA), Deutsche Gesellschaft für Technische Zusammenarbeit (GTZ), Germany, and the Department for International Development (DFID), United Kingdom. Throughout its two-year life, the JLI received the unstinting support of the World Health Organization and the World Bank.

With the publication of the JLI Strategy Report, momentum behind the JLI is being channeled into strengthening existing groups and a JLI-successor initiative to maintain independent perspectives and to promote JLI recommendations. This alliance for action will seek to advance learning in the field, advocate for the importance of learning in the field, and enhance the effectiveness of all actors in human resources for health.

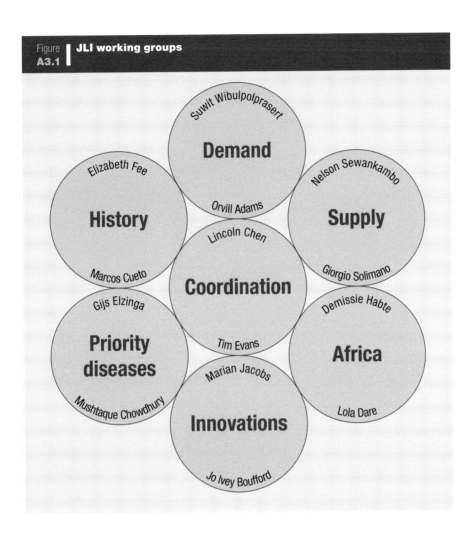

Figure A3.1 | JLI working groups

Suwit Wibulpolprasert

Demand

Orvill Adams

Elizabeth Fee

History

Marcos Cueto

Nelson Sewankambo

Supply

Giorgio Solimano

Lincoln Chen

Coordination

Tim Evans

Gijs Elzinga

Priority diseases

Mushtaque Chowdhury

Demissie Habte

Africa

Lola Dare

Marian Jacobs

Innovations

Jo Ivey Boufford

JLI working groups

Coordination – To facilitate the efforts of all the working groups, to promote the joint learning process with an emphasis on cross-cutting issues, and to undertake the necessary research, writing, and production of an evidence-based advocacy and strategy report

Co-chairs: Lincoln Chen, Harvard University, USA

Tim Evans, World Health Organization, Switzerland

Demand – To analyze the landscape of the demand side of the health workforce and to formulate policy options for the improvement of human resource management in support of more equitable, efficient and better quality health

Co-chairs   Orvill Adams, World Health Organization, Switzerland

Suwit Wibulpolprasert, Ministry of Public Health, Thailand

Supply – To landscape the mechanisms and modalities of education and training and to recommend strategies for greater relevance, innovation, and equity in the production of the health workforce

Co-chairs   Nelson Sewankambo, Makerere University, Uganda
Giorgio Solimano, University of Chile, Chile

Africa – To map the current landscape of human resources for health in Africa, to identify key issues, and to define a broad strategy to address the prevailing workforce crisis

Co-chairs   Lola Dare, Center for Health Science Training, Research and Development International, Nigeria
Demissie Habte, BRAC School of Public Health, Bangladesh

Priority diseases – To analyze the current and future needs for human resources to fight select diseases, using supply and demand lens to explore new models for control within an integrated health system

Co-chairs   Mushtaque Chowdhury, BRAC, Bangladesh, and Columbia University, USA
Gijs Elzinga, National Institute of Public Health and Environment, The Netherlands

Innovations – To learn about innovative approaches to leadership development and human resource capacity development for health

Co-chairs   Jo Ivey Boufford, New York University: The Wagner School of Public Service, USA
Marian Jacobs, University of Cape Town, South Africa

History – To illuminate historical lessons on human resources for health and development

Co-chairs   Elizabeth Fee, National Library of Medicine: National Institutes of Health, USA
Marcos Cueto, Universidad Peruana Cayetano Heredia, Peru

Gender task force – To develop an evidence base and advocacy strategy around identifying the gender dimensions of the health workforce in an effort to improve strategies for strengthening human resources for health.

Co-chairs   Hilary Brown, World Health Organization, Switzerland
Laura Reichenbach, Harvard Center for Population and Development Studies, USA

JLI secretariat

The Joint Learning Initiative was supported and coordinated by a secretariat comprising:

Rockefeller Foundation	Hilary Brown	
	Vasant Narasimhan	
JSI Research & Training Institute	Matt Habinowski	
	Alec McKinney	
	Betsy Nesbitt	
Harvard Global Equity Initiative	Piya Hanvoravongchai	Victoria Manuelli
	Swathi Kappagantula	Sarah Michael
	Carol Kotilainen	Vasant Narasimhan
	Christopher Linnane	Jonathan Welch

The JLI report

The JLI Report was produced under the direction of Lincoln C. Chen and coordinated by Sarah Michael and Piya Hanvoravongchai. The core report team consisted of the following members:

Research and writing	Sudhir Anand	Christoph Kurowski
	Lincoln C. Chen	Sarah Michael
	Alex de Waal	Fitzhugh Mullan
	Delanyo Dovlo	Barbara Stilwell
	Gilles Dussault	Jonathan Welch
	Piya Hanvoravongchai	
Research support	Till Baernighausen	Swathi Kappagantula
	Shashank Goel	Victoria Manuelli
	Celina Gorre	Elizabeth McCarthy
Translation of the executive summary	Marcos Cueto (Spanish)	
	Gilles Dussault (French)	

Other research and writing contributors to the report include:
Orvill Adams, Bruce Aylward, Jo Ivey Boufford, Peter G. Bourne, Hilary Brown, Theodore Brown, Mushtaque Chowdhury, Marcos Cueto, Khassoum Diallo, Ed Elmendorf, Gijs Elzinga, Timothy Evans, Elizabeth Fee, Gebre Tsadkan Gebretensae, Pat Hughes, Jeremy Hurst, Ingo Imhoff, Marian Jacobs, Stephen Kinoti, Riitta-Liisa Kolehmainen-Aitken, Uta Lehmann, Tim Martineau, Inke Mathauer, Hugo Mercer, Catherine Michaud, Sigrun Mogedal, Vasant Narasimhan, Sidney Ndeki, John Norcini, Mary O'Neil, Andrea Pantoja, Gail Reed, Nelson Sewankambo, Steven Simoens, Giorgio Solimano, Suwit Wibulpolprasert, Rony Zachariah

Administrative support	Carol Kotilainen
	Christopher Linnane
	Staff, Harvard Global Equity Initiative

Editing and production	Meta de Coquereaumont
	Mary Goundrey
	Thomas Roncoli
	Bruce Ross-Larson
	Christopher Trott
	Timothy Walker
	Elaine Wilson
	Communications Development Incorporated

Partners and donors

The Atlantic Philanthropies (USA), Inc.
Bill & Melinda Gates Foundation
Canadian International Development Agency
Department for International Development, United Kingdom
Deutsche Gesellschaft für Technische Zusammenarbeit, Germany
Global Equity Initiative, Harvard University
JSI Research & Training Institute, Inc.
Open Society Institute
The Rockefeller Foundation
Swedish Sida
World Health Organization
World Bank

JLI working group members

Coordination

Orvill Adams	World Health Organization, Switzerland
Jo Ivey Boufford	New York University: The Wagner School of Public Service, USA
Lincoln Chen	Harvard University, USA
Mushtaque Chowdhury	BRAC, Bangladesh, and Columbia University, USA
Marcos Cueto	Universidad Peruana Cayetano Heredia, Peru
Lola Dare	Center for Health Science Training, Research and Development International, Nigeria
Gilles Dussault	World Bank Institute, USA
Gijs Elzinga	National Institute of Public Health and the Environment, The Netherlands

Tim Evans	World Health Organization, Switzerland
Elizabeth Fee	National Library of Medicine: National Institutes of Health, USA
Demissie Habte	BRAC School of Public Health, Bangladesh
Marian Jacobs	University of Cape Town, South Africa
Joel Lamstein	JSI Research & Training Institute, Inc., USA
Anders Nordstrom	World Health Organization, Switzerland
Ariel Pablos-Mendez	World Health Organization, Switzerland
William Pick	University of Witwatersrand School of Public Health, South Africa
Nelson Sewankambo	Makerere University, Uganda
Giorgio Solimano	University of Chile, Chile
Suwit Wibulpolprasert	Ministry of Public Health, Thailand

Demand

Orvill Adams	World Health Organization, Switzerland
Frances Brebner	Department of Health, Samoa
James Buchan	Queen Margaret University College, United Kingdom
Delanyo Dovlo	Ministry of Health, Ghana
Akram Eltom	International Organization of Migration, Switzerland
Timothy Evans	World Health Organization, Switzerland
Paulo Ferrinho	Garcia de Orta Association for Development and Cooperation, Portugal
Thomas Hall	University of California at San Francisco, USA
Piya Hanvoravongchai	International Health Policy Program, Thailand
Pintusorn Hempisut	Ministry of Public Health, Thailand
Riita-Liisa Kolehmainen-Aitken	Management Sciences for Health, USA
Gustavo Nigenda	National Institute of Public Health, Mexico
Judith Oulton	International Council of Nurses, Switzerland
Alex Preker	World Bank, USA
David Sanders	University of the Western Cape: School of Public Health, South Africa
Agus Suwandono	Ministry of Health, Indonesia
Suwit Wibulpolprasert	Ministry of Public Health, Thailand
Christiane Wiskow	International Labour Organization, Switzerland

Supply

Mushtaque Chowdhury	BRAC, Bangladesh and Columbia University, USA
Ed Elmendorf	World Bank (retired), USA
Charles Godue	Pan American Health Organization, USA
Gerald Majoor	Maastricht University, The Netherlands
Hugo Mercer	World Health Organization, Switzerland

Peter Ndumbe	University of Yaounde, Cameroon
Andrzej Rys	Krakow School of Public Health, Poland
Nelson Sewankambo	Makerere University, Uganda
Giorgio Solimano	University of Chile, Chile
Kunaviktikul Wipada	Changmai University, Thailand

Africa

Eric Buch	University of Pretoria, South Africa
Rufaro Chatora	WHO/AFRO, Congo
Abdallah Daar	University of Toronto: Joint Center for Bioethics, Canada
Delanyo Dovlo	Ministry of Health, Ghana
Mario Fresta	Ministry of Health, Angola
Akpa Gbary	WHO/AFRO, Congo
Demisse Habte	BRAC School of Public Health, Bangladesh
Carel Ijsselmuiden	University of Pretoria, South Africa
Uta Lehman	University of Western Cape: School of Public Health, South Africa
Tim Martineau	Liverpool School of Tropical Medicine, United Kingdom
Olive Munjanja	Commonwealth Secretariat, Tanzania
Vasant Narasimhan	McKinsey & Co, USA
Peter Ndumbe	University of Yaounde, Cameroon
David Sanders	University of Western Cape: School of Public Health, South Africa

Priority diseases

Juan Jose Amador	Ministry of Health, Nicaragua
Bruce Aylward	World Health Organization, Switzerland
Raj Bahn	All India Institute of Medical Sciences, India
Leo Blanc	World Health Organization, Switzerland
Mushtaque Chowdhury	BRAC, Bangladesh and Columbia University, USA
Marjolein Dieleman	Royal Tropical Institute, The Netherlands
Gilles Dussault	World Bank Institute, USA
Gijs Elzinga	National Institute of Public Health and the Environment, The Netherlands
Jeremy Farrar	Oxford University Clinical Research Unit, Vietnam
Eva Harris	University of California at Berkeley, USA
Anne Mills	London School of Hygiene and Tropical Medicine, United Kingdom
Vinand Nantulya	Global Fund for HIV/AIDS, Tuberculosis, and Malaria, Switzerland

Margie Peden	World Health Organization, Switzerland
Mark Rosenberg	Task Force for Child Survival and Development, USA
Robert Scherpbier	World Health Organization, Switzerland

Innovations

F. H. Abed	BRAC, Bangladesh
Don Berwick	Institute for Healthcare Improvement, USA
Silvia Bino	Insitute of Public Health, Albania
Jo Ivey Boufford	New York University: The Wagner School of Public Service, USA
David Bradley	The Advisory Board, USA
Hilary Brown	World Health Organization, Switzerland
Francisco Campos	Universidade Federal de Minas Gerais, Brazil
Abdallah Daar	University of Toronto: Joint Center for Bioethics, Canada
Lola Dare	Center for Health Science Training, Research and Development International, Nigeria
Bill Drayton	Ashoka, USA
Judy Hargadon	Changing Workforce Program, United Kingdom
Marian Jacobs	University of Cape Town, South Africa
Dan Kaseje	Tropical Institute of Community Health and Development in Africa, Kenya
Mary Ann Lansang	INCLEN, Philippines
Daniel Lopez-Acuna	Pan American Health Organization, USA
Jose State Noronha	University of Rio de Janeiro, Brazil
Ariel Pablos-Mendez	World Health Organization, Switzerland
Jawaya Small	University of Cape Town: School of Public Health, South Africa
Suwit Wibulpolprasert	Ministry of Public Health, Thailand
James Wilk	Interchange Research, Canada

History

Giovanni Berlinguer	Comitato Nazionale per la Bioetica, Italy
Sanjoy Bhattacharya	University College London: The Wellcome Trust Centre for the History of Medicine, United Kingdom
Anne-Emanuelle Birn	New School University: Milano Graduate School, USA
Theodore Brown	University of Rochester: Department of History, USA
Marcos Cueto	Universidad Peruana Cayetano Heredia, Peru
Bernardino Fantini	University of Geneva: Institut d'Histoire de la Médecine et de la Santé, Switzerland

Elizabeth Fee	National Library of Medicine: National Institutes of Health, USA
Stephen Kunitz	University of Rochester Medical Center, USA
Nisia Lima	Trinidad Casa Oswaldo Cruz, Brazil
Socrates Litsios	World Health Organization (retired), Switzerland
Maryinez Lyons	International Organization for Migration, Kenya
Eiji Marui	Juntendo University Medical School: Department of Public Health, Japan
Anne-Marie Moulin	Institut de Recherche pour le Developpement Societé et Santé, France
William Muraskin	Queens College, USA
Mary Northridge	American Journal of Public Health, Columbia University, USA
Ariel Pablos-Mendez	World Health Organization, Switzerland
Randall Packard	The Johns Hopkins University, USA
William Pick	University of Witwatersrand: School of Public Health, South Africa
Yogan Pillay	The Equity Project, South Africa
Emilio Quevedo	Universidad Nacional de Colombia: Facultad de Medicina, Colombia
Julia Royall	National Library of Medicine: National Institutes of Health, USA
Darwin Stapleton	The Rockefeller Archive, USA
Simon Szreter	St. John's College, Cambridge, United Kingdom

Publications Committee

| Theodore Brown | University of Rochester Medical Center, USA |
| Mary Northridge | American Journal of Public Health, Columbia University, USA |

Gender task force

Sudhir Anand	Global Equity Initiative, Harvard University, USA
Rebecka O. Alffram	Sida, Sweden
Hilary Brown	World Health Organization, Switzerland
Lincoln Chen	Global Equity Initiative, Harvard University, USA
Lola Dare	Center for Health Science Training, Research and Development International, Nigeria
Claudia Garcia-Morena	World Health Organization, Switzerland
Anwar Islam	Canadian International Development Agency, Canada
Churnrurtai Kanchanachitra	Institute for Population and Social Research, Mahidol University, Thailand

Riitta-Liisa Kolehmainen-Aitken Management Sciences for Health, USA
Mariana López Ortega Fundación Mexicana para la Salud, Mexico
Piroska Ostlin National Institute of Public Health, Sweden
Laura Reichenbach Harvard Center for Population and Development Studies, USA
Pia Rockhold The Ministry of Foreign Affairs, Denmark
Hilary Standing Institute of Development Studies, University of Sussex, United Kingdom

JLI publications

Working group reports
Report of the Demand Working Group
    Papers will be published by the Human Resources for Health Online Journal
Report of the Supply Working Group
Report of the Africa Working Group
Report of the Select Priority Diseases Working Group
    Papers will be published by the *Bulletin* of WHO
Report of the History Working Group
    Papers will be published in the American Journal of Public Health
Gender Task Force
    Forthcoming volume on Gender and the Global Health Workforce

Working papers

Agble, Rosanna, Frank Nyonator, Carmen Casanovas, and Robert Scherpbier. 2004. "Case Study: Ghana Experience on Human Resources to Implement the Infant and Young Child Feeding Strategy." Ghana Health Service, Ghana.

Alkire, Sabina, and Lincoln Chen. 2004. "Medical Exceptionalism in International Migration: Should Doctors and Nurses Be Treated Differently?" The Joint Learning Initiative, Human Resources for Health, and The Global Equity Initiative, Harvard University Asia Center, USA.

Anand, Sudhir, and Till Baernighausen. 2004. "Human Resources and Health Outcomes." Global Equity Initiative, USA, and Oxford University, United Kingdom.

Bhattacharya, Sanjoy. 2004. "Uncertain Advances: A Review of the Final Phases of the Smallpox Eradication Programme in India, 1960–1980." The Wellcome Trust Centre for the History of Medicine, United Kingdom.

Birn, Anne-Emanuelle. 2004. "Going Global: Uruguay, Child Well-being and International Health, 1890–1940." University of Toronto, Canada.

Boufford, Jo Ivey. 2004. "Leadership for Global Health." New York University: The Wagner School of Public Service, USA.

Buchan, James, Tina Parkin, and Julie Sochalski. 2003. "International Nurse Mobility: Trends and Policy Implications." Queen Margaret University College, United Kingdom and University of Pennsylvania, USA.

Cash, Richard. 2004. "Ethical Issues for Manpower Development." Harvard School of Public Health, USA.

Cash, Richard. 2004. "Strengthening Research Capacity in Developing Countries through Manpower Development: A Brief Examination of Opportunities and Impediments." Harvard School of Public Health, USA.

Campos, Francisco, José Roberto Ferreira, Maria Fátima de Souza, Raphael Augusto Teixeira de Aguiar. 2004. "The Innovations on Human Resources Development and the Role of Community Health Workers." Universidade Federal de Minas Gerais Núcleo de Pesquisa em Saúde Coletiva, Brazil.

Chowdhury, Mushtaque. 2003. "Health Workforce for TB Control by DOTS: The BRAC Case." BRAC, Bangladesh.

Cueto, Marcos. 2004. "The Origins of Primary Health Care and Selective Primary Health Care." Universidad Peruana Cayetano Heredia, Peru.

Dare, Lola. "The Alternate Workforce: Involving Communities in Priority Health Problems." Center for Health Science Training, Research and Development International, Nigeria.

de Leonardis, Ota. 2004. "Social Capital, Sociability and Health." University of Sociology and Social Research, Italy.

Dovlo, Delanyo, and Tim Martineau. 2004. "Review of Evidence for Push and Pull Factors and Impact on Health Worker Mobility in Africa." Ministry of Health, Ghana and Liverpool School of Tropical Medicine, United Kingdom.

Dovlo, Delanyo. 2004. "Assessing HRH Wastage and Improving Staff Retention: An African Perspective." Ministry of Health, Ghana.

Estévez, Rafael, Oscar Arteaga, and Giorgio Solimano. 2004. "Building Human Resource Capability for Health." TOP Consultores SA, Chile, University of Chile, Chile.

Farrar, Jeremy, and Eva Harris. 2004. "Dengue Fever/Malaria Case Study." Oxford University Clinical Research Unit, Vietnam and University of California at Berkeley, USA.

Fee, Elizabeth, Theodore Brown, and Marcos Cueto. 2004. "The World Health Organization and the Transition from 'International' to 'Global' Public Health." National Library of Medicine: National Institutes of Health, USA; University of Rochester, USA; Universidad Peruana Cayetano Heredia, Peru.

Ferrinho, Paulo, Wim Van Lerberghe, Inês Fronteira, Fátima Hipólito Ba Soc, and André Biscaia. 2004. "Dual Practice in the Health Sector: Review of the Evidence." Garcia de Orta Development and Cooperation Association, Portugal; World Health Association, Switzerland.

Glenngård, Anna, and Anders Anell. 2003. "Investment in Human Resources for Health—Problems, Approaches and Donor Experiences." The Swedish Institute for Health Economics, Sweden.

Happiness, Osegie, Taiwo Adewole, Olamide Bandele. "Brain Drain and Human Resource Development in Nigeria." Center for Health Science Training, Research and Development International, Nigeria, and National Institute for Medical Research, Nigeria.

Hargadon, Judy and Paul Plsek. 2004. "Complexity and Health Workforce Issues." New Ways of Working Modernisation Agency, United Kingdom; Paul E. Plsek & Associates, United Kingdom.

Harries, Tony, Felix Salaniponi, Rony Zachariah, Karin Bergstrom, Gijs Elzinga. 2004. "Human Resources for Control of Tuberculosis and HIV-Associated Tuberculosis: Unresolved Issues." National TB Control Programme, Lilongwe, Malawi; National Institute for Public Health & the Environment, The Netherlands; Médecins Sans Frontières, Belgium; World Health Organization, Switzerland.

Kanyesigye, Edward and Ssendyona, G. M. 2003. "Payment of Lunch Allowance: A Case Study of the Uganda Health Service." Ministry of Health, Uganda; Ministry of Public Service, Uganda.

Kaseje, Dan. 2004. "Community Involvement in Health Professionals' Education to Strengthen Them for their Role in Strengthening Health Care Systems in Africa." The Tropical Institute of Community Health and Development, Kenya.

Kolehmainen-Aitken, Riitta-Liisa. 2003. "Decentralization's Impact on the Health Workforce: Perspective of Managers, Workers and National Leaders." Management Sciences for Health, USA.

Kunaviktikul, Wipada, Suparat Wangsrikhun, Petsunee Tungcharernkul, Wichit Srisuphun, Lui Ming, Nuthamon Vuthanon. 2004. "Training of Human Resources for Health: An Integrative Literature Review." Changmai University, Thailand.

Kunitz, Stephen J. 2004. "The Making and Breaking of Federated Yugoslavia, and Its Impact on Health." University of Rochester School of Medicine and Dentistry, USA.

Kurowski, Christoph. 2004. "Scope, Characteristics and Policy Implications of the Health Worker Shortage in Low-Income Countries of Sub-Saharan Africa." World Bank, USA.

Lehmann, Uta, Irwin Friedman, and David Sanders. 2004. "Review of the Utilisation and Effectiveness of Community-Based Health Workers in Africa." University of the Western Cape, South Africa; SEED Trust, South Africa.

Lethbridge, Elizabeth Jane. 2003. "Public Sector Reform and HRH Demand." Public Services International Research Unit, United Kingdom.

Lima, Nísia Trinidade. 2004. "Public Health and Social Ideas in Modern Brazil." Fundação Oswaldo Cruz—FIOCRUZ, Brazil.

Litsios, Socrates. 2004. "The Christian Medical Commission and the Development of WHO's Primary Heath Care Approach." World Health Organization, Switzerland.

Lyons, Maryinez. "Health Workers in Uganda: From Crisis to Crisis." International Organization for Migration, Kenya.

Majoor, Gerard. 2003. "Recent Innovations in Education of Human Resources for Health." Maastricht University, The Netherlands.

Muraskin, William. 2004. "The Global Alliance for Vaccines and Immunization (GAVI): Is It a New Model for Effective Public Private Cooperation in International Public Health?" Queens College, USA.

Naga, Ramses Abul, and Hugo Mercer. 2004. "Stakeholders' Opinions on Priorities in Human Resources for Health." World Health Organization, Switzerland; University of Lausanne, Switzerland.

Ndumbe, Peter. 2004. "The Training of Human Resources for Health in Africa." University of Yaounde, Cameroon.

Neufeld, Vic and Nancy Johnson. 2004. "Training and Development of Health Leaders." McMaster University, Canada.

Nigenda, Gustavo, José Arturo Ruiz, and Rosa Bejarano. 2004. "The Wastage of Doctors in Mexico: Towards the Construction of a Common Methodology." Mexican Health Foundation, Mexico.

Pablos-Mendez, Ariel, and Hilary Brown. 2004. "Knowledge Management in Public Health." World Health Organization, Switzerland and the Rockefeller Foundation, USA.

Preker, Alex, Jan Ruthkowski, Doug Smith, Christoph Kurowski, Marko Vujicic, and Richard Scheffler. 2004. "Impact of Globalization and Macro Economic Policies on Health Care Labor Markets." World Bank, USA, World Health Organization, Switzerland, and the London School of Hygiene and Tropical Medicine, United Kingdom.

Quevedo, Emilio. 2004. "International Interests and Local Negotiation: The Rockefeller Foundation, Hookworm Disease and Latin America." National University of Colombia, Colombia.

Reichenbach, Laura and Brown, Hilary. 2004. "Gender and Academic Medicine: Impacts on the Health Workforce." Harvard Center for Population and Development Studies, USA and The Rockefeller Foundation, USA. Forthcoming in BMJ 2004.

Rigoli, Félix, and Oscar Arteaga. 2004. "The Experience of the Latin America and Caribbean Observatory of Human Resources in Health." Pan American Health Organization, USA; Universidad de Chile, Chile.

Stapleton, Darwin. 2004. "Fellowships and Field Stations: The Globalization of Public Health Knowledge, 1920–1950." Rockefeller Archive Center, USA.

Talbot, Yves, Niall Byrne, Monica Riutort, Silvia Takeda, and Luis Fernando Rolim Sampaio. 2003. "Primary Health Care in the Americas: Problems and Challenges in Developing Primary Health Care Professionals." University of Toronto, Canada and Grupo Hospitalar Conceicao, Brazil.

Wahba, Jackline. 2004. "Health Labour Markets: Incentives or Institutions?" University of Southampton, United Kingdom.

Wibulpolprasert, Suwit, Siriwan Pitayarangsarit, and Pintusorn Hempisut. 2003. "International Service Trade and Its Implication on Human Resources for Health: A Case Study of Thailand." Health Systems Research Institute, Thailand; Ministry of Public Health, Thailand.

JLI meetings and consultations

2002

February 1. Addis-Ababa, Ethiopia. World Bank/AFRO Conference where HRH needs and opportunities were discussed

September 23–24. New York, USA. Rockefeller Foundation consultation on *Problem-Solving Capacity for Priority Diseases of the Poor*

October 2. Zagreb, Croatia. JLI preliminary consultation with members of European schools of public health

November 15–16. Arusha, Tanzania. First JLI co-chair consultation, including exchanges with African participants attending Forum for Health Research

2003

January 23–24. Stockholm, Sweden. Consultative session hosted by Sida to develop concept and operations of JLI

March 27–29. Cape Town, South Africa. Major JLI co-chair consultation, including Working Group Africa and Working Group Innovation meetings

April 22–22. New York, USA. Working Group Supply planning meeting

May 8–10. Veyrier-du-Lac, France. Working Group Demand meeting

May 19–20. Oxford, United Kingdom. JLI preparatory session on scientific challenges in producing Strategy Report

May 28. Cambridge, USA. JLI consultation on potential writers, authors, and contributors to JLI Report

June 9–13. Rajendrapur, Bangladesh. Working Group Coordination meeting

July 29. Brasilia, Brazil. Working Group Coordination meeting

September 19. Tblisi, Georgia. JLI informal consultation on *A Public Health Leadership Network*

Sept. 29–Oct. 1. Accra, Ghana. Working Group Africa meeting

October 23–24. London, United Kingdom. Working Group Coordination meeting

Oct. 27–Nov. 1. Bellagio, Italy. Working Group History meeting

Oct. 30–Nov. 1. London, United Kingdom. Working Group Supply meeting

November 11–12. Naarden, The Netherlands. Working Group Priority Diseases meeting

December 8. London, United Kingdom. Working Group Innovation consultation on *Complexity Theory and Human Resources*

December 9–12. Bellagio, Italy. Working Group Coordination meeting

2004

February 2–4. Chonburi, Thailand. Working Group Demand workshop

February 13. Kaunas, Lithuania. JLI consultation on *The Development of an Effective Health Sector Workforce Among Eastern European Countries*

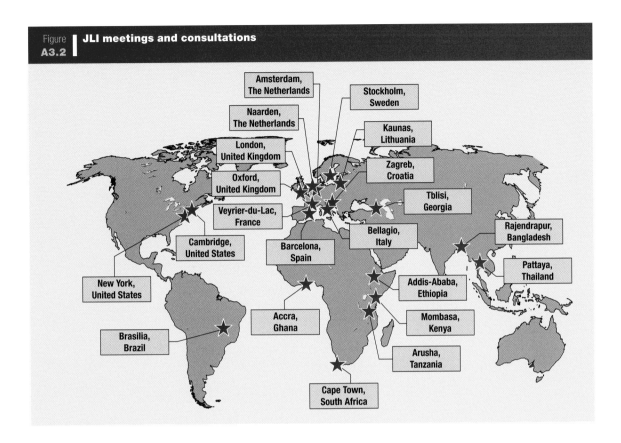

Figure A3.2 — JLI meetings and consultations

Amsterdam, The Netherlands

Stockholm, Sweden

Naarden, The Netherlands

Kaunas, Lithuania

London, United Kingdom

Zagreb, Croatia

Oxford, United Kingdom

Tblisi, Georgia

Veyrier-du-Lac, France

Bellagio, Italy

Rajendrapur, Bangladesh

Cambridge, United States

Barcelona, Spain

Pattaya, Thailand

New York, United States

Addis-Ababa, Ethiopia

Accra, Ghana

Mombasa, Kenya

Brasilia, Brazil

Arusha, Tanzania

Cape Town, South Africa

March 11–12. Barcelona, Spain. Working Group Innovations meeting

March 15–16. Barcelona, Spain. Working Group Coordination meeting

May 21–2. London, United Kingdom. JLI consultation on *The Gender Dimensions of the Global Health Workforce*

May 27–28. Amsterdam, The Netherlands. Working Group Select Priority Diseases: The Netherlands Round Table on *Vertical Program Contribution to Health System Strengthening*

May 31–June 2. Mombasa, Kenya. Working Group Africa meeting

June 11–13. Stockholm, Sweden. JLI–WHO–Institute Future Studies workshop on *International Migration*

August 11–13. Brasilia, Brazil. Brazil Country HRH Consultation

September 5–8. Cape Town, South Africa. South African national consultation on human resources for health and JLI working group coordination meeting; WHO workshop on a global research agenda for human resources in health and WHO/World Bank/JLI preparation for the December 2004 High Level Forum in Abuja

JLI participants

The work of the Joint Learning Initiative was supported by many individuals, institutions, and organizations, representing a wide range of interests, concerns, and expertise. To all those who provided insights, support, and commitment to the strengthening of the JLI work on human resources for health, we express our gratitude and thanks.

F. H. Abed	BRAC, Bangladesh
Theodor Abelin	World Federation of Public Health Associations, Switzerland
Orvill Adams	World Health Organization, Switzerland
Taiwo Adewole	CHESTRAD, Nigeria
Rosanna Agble	Nutrition Unit, Ghana
Carlos Agudelo	ACOESP, Columbia
Rebecka Alffram	Sida, Sweden
Juan Jose Amador	Ministry of Health, Nicaragua
Sudhir Anand	Global Equity Initiative, Harvard University, USA
Douglas Angus	MHA Program, School of Management, Canada
Maru Aregawi	World Health Organization, Switzerland
Haroutune Armenian	American University of Armenia, Armenia
Juan Arroyo	Universidad Peruana Cayetano Heredia, Peru
Oscar Herrara Arteaga	Universidad de Chile: School of Public Health, Chile
Annella Auer	Pan American Health Organization, USA
Magda Awases	World Health Organization–AFRO, Congo
Bruce Aylward	World Health Organization, Switzerland
Mashbadrakh Baasanjav	Mongolian Foundation for Open Society, Mongolia
Till Baernighausen	Harvard School of Public Health, USA
Raj Bahn	All India Institute of Medical Sciences, India
Brendan Bain	Department of Community Health and Psychiatry UWI, Jamaica
Peter Barron	Health System Trust, South Africa
Jose Barzelatto	Center for Health and Social Policy, USA
Mary Bassett	New York City Department of Health and Mental Hygiene, USA
Jacques Baudouy	World Bank, USA
Robert Beaglehole	World Health Organization, Switzerland
Mike Bennish	Indepth Africa, South Africa
Karin Bergstrom	World Health Organization, Switzerland
Giovanni Berlinguer	Comitato Nazionale per la Bioetica, Italy
Don Berwick	Institute for Healthcare Improvement, USA
Helen Bevan	NHS Modernization Agency, United Kingdom
Sanjoy Bhattacharya	The Wellcome Trust, United Kingdom

Silvia Bino	Institute of Public Health, Albania
Anne-Emanuelle Birn	Department of Public Health, Canada
Leo Blanc	World Health Organization, Switzerland
Patrick Bond	University of Witwatersrand, South Africa
R. Borroto	Escuela de Salud Publica de Cuba, Cuba
Jo Ivey Boufford	New York University: The Wagner School of Public Service, USA
Frances Brebner	Department of Health, Samoa, USA
Marc Brodin	Départment de Santé Publique, France
Hilary Brown	World Health Organization, Switzerland
Theodore Brown	The University of Rochester Medical Center, USA
Eric Buch	University of Pretoria, South Africa
James Buchan	Queen Margaret University College, United Kingdom
Jacques Bury	Sanitaire Qualitative IMSP, Switzerland
Pruscia Buscell	The Plexus Institute, USA
Richard Cash	Harvard School of Public Health, USA
Luisa Castillo	Instituto Altos Estudios en Salud Publica, Venezuela
Rufaro Chatora	World Health Organization: AFRO, Congo
Lincoln Chen	Global Equity Initiative, Harvard University, USA
Vichai Chokewiwat	Ministry of Public Health, Thailand
Mushtaque Chowdhury	BRAC, Bangladesh and Columbia University, USA
Laurence Codjia	CESAG, Senegal
Maria Coll-Seck	Ministry of Health, Senegal
Marcos Cueto	Instituto de Estudios Peruanos, Peru
Abdallah Daar	University of Toronto: Joint Center for Bioethics, Canada
Mario Dal Poz	World Health Organization, Switzerland
Isabel d'Almeida	Ministry of Health, Guinea-Bissau
John Darrah	Private consultant, USA
Naomar de Almeida	Universidad de Bahia, Brasil
Shanta Devarajan	World Bank, USA
Alex de Waal	Justice Africa, United Kingdom
Marjolein Dieleman	Koninklijk Instituut vor de Tropen (KIT), The Netherlands
Carmen Dolea	World Health Organization, Switzerland
Delanyo Dovlo	Ministry of Health, Ghana
Leslie Doyal	University of Bristol: Social Science Complex, United Kingdom
Bill Drayton	Ashoka, USA
Norbert Dreesch	World Health Organization, Switzerland
Nel Druce	DFID Health Systems Resource Centre, United Kingdom

Yongon Dungu	Public Health Association of Mongolia, Mongolia
Gilles Dussault	World Bank Institute, USA
Sadikova Dzhamilya	The Soros Foundation, Kazakhstan
Francisco de Campos	Federal University of Minas Gerais, Portugal
A. M. El Hassan	Institute of Endemic Diseases, Sudan
Ed Elmendorf	World Bank, USA
Akram Eltom	International Organization Migration, Switzerland
Gijs Elzinga	National Institute of Public Health and the Environment, The Netherlands
Rafael Estevez	Top Consultores, Chile
David Evans	World Health Organization, Switzerland
Timothy Evans	World Health Organization, Switzerland
Bernardino Fantini	Institut d'Histoire de la Medecine et de la Sante, Switzerland
Jeremy Farrar	Oxford University Clinical Research Unit, Viet Nam
Elizabeth Fee	National Library of Medicine: National Institutes of Health, USA
Ana Ferrari	Maria Universidad de la Republica, Uruguay
Paulo Ferrinho	Association for Development and Cooperation, Portugal
Laura Feuerwerker	Associacao Brasileira de Educacao Medica, Brazil
David Fleming	Bill and Melinda Gates Foundation, USA
Helga Fogstad	World Health Organization, Switzerland
Beverly Freeman	Private Consultant, USA
Mario Fresta	Ministry of Health of Nicaragua, Nicaragua
Inês Fronteira	Association for Development and Cooperation, Portugal
Hector Gallardo	City Hospital of Guadalajara, Mexico
Claudia Garcia-Morena	World Health Organization, Switzerland
Akpa Gbary	World Health Organization–AFRO, Congo
Christian Gericke	Technische Universitat Berlin, Germany
Sholom Glouberman	Baycrest Centre for Geriatric Care, Canada
Charles Godue	Pan American Health Organization, USA
G. Gonzalez-Echeverria	National School of Public Health, Colombia
Matt Habinowski	JSI Research & Training Institute, Inc., USA
Demissie Habte	BRAC School of Public Health, Bangladesh
Thomas Hall	University of California at San Francisco, USA
Piya Hanvoravongchai	International Health Policy Program, Thailand and Global Equity Initiative, Harvard University, USA
Osegie Happiness	CHESTRAD, Nigeria
Judy Hargadon	New Ways of Working Modernization Agency, United Kingdom

Anthony Harries	British High Commission, Malawi
Eva Harris	University of California at Berkeley, USA
Jane Haycock	DFID, United Kingdom
Petra Heitkamp	World Health Organization, Switzerland
Pintusorn Hempisuth	Ministry of Public Health, Thailand
Cossa Humberto	Ministry of Health, Mozambique
Jussi Huttunen	National Public Health Institute of Finland, Finland
Carel Ijsselmuden	University of Pretoria, South Africa and COHRED, Switzerland
Ingo Imhoff	GTZ International Cooperation and Programs, Germany
Anwar Islam	Canadian International Development Agency, Canada
Iskandar Ismailov	OSI Assistance Foundation, Uzbekistan
Marian Jacobs	University of Cape Town: Child Health Unit, South Africa
Edgar Jarillo	Maestria en Medicina, Mexico
Givi Javashvili	National Health Institute, Georgia
David Johnson	IHSD, United Kingdom
Calestous Juma	Harvard University, USA
Churnrurtai Kanchanachitra	Institute for Population and Social Research, Thailand
Anna-Carin Kandimaa	Sida, Swedish Embassy, Zambia
Edward Kanyesigye	Uganda Ministry of Health, Uganda
Swathi Kappagantula	Global Equity Initiative, Harvard University, USA
Dan Kaseje	Tropical Institute of Community Health and Development in Africa, Kenya
Arthur Kauffman	University of New Mexico, USA
Stuart Kaufman	Bios Group LP, USA
Ilona Kickbusch	Pan American Health Organization, USA
Stephen Kinoti	SARA/AED/USAID, USA
Daniel Klass	University of Winnipeg, Canada
Richard Kohl	Consultant, USA
Riita-Liisa Kolehmainen-Aitken	Management Sciences for Health, USA
Wipada Kunaviktikul	Chiang Mai University, Thailand
Stephen Kunitz	University of Rochester Medical Center, USA
Rolf Korte	GTZ, Germany
Luka Kovacic	University of Zagreb School of Public Health, Croatia
Christoph Kurowski	World Bank, USA
Joel Lamstein	JSI Research & Training Institute, Inc., USA
Mary Ann Lansang	INCLEN/Philippines, Philippines
Robert Lawrence	Johns Hopkins Bloomberg School of Public Health, USA

Uta Lehmann	University of Western Cape: School of Public Health, South Africa
Ota Leonardis	De Dipartimento di Sociologia e Ricerca Sociale, Italy
Maureen Lewis	Center for Global Development, USA
Jane Lethbridge	Public Services International Research United, United Kingdom
Paul Light	C. Robert F. Wagner School of Public Health, USA
Nisia Lima	FIOCRUZ, Brazil
Jennifer Linkins	World Health Organization, Switzerland
Socrates Litsios	World Health Organization, Switzerland
Julian Lob-Levyt	UNAIDS, Switzerland
Knut Lonnroth	World Health Organization: Stop TB Program, Switzerland
Daniel Lopez-Acuna	Pan American Health Organization, USA
Jorge Lossio	University of Manchester, United Kingdom
Frank Lostumbo	American Public Health Association, USA
Rene Lowenson	TARSC, Zimbabwe
Maryinez Lyons	International Organization for Migration, Kenya
Sarah Macfarlane	The Rockefeller Foundation, USA
Gudjón Magnússon	World Health Organization, Denmark
Gerard Majoor	Institute of Medical Education, The Netherlands
José Martin-Moreno	Maria Ministerio de Sanidad y Consumo, Spain
Tim Martineau	Liverpool School of Tropical Medicine, United Kingdom
Eiji Marui	Juntendo University Medical School, Japan
Rashad Massoud	Quality Assurance Project, USA
Inke Mathauer	GTZ, Germany
Clare Matterson	The Wellcome Trust: Medicine, Society and History Division, United Kingdom
Princess Matwa	University of the Western Cape, South Africa
Alan Maynard	University of York, United Kingdom
Lucia Mazarrasa	Ministerio de Sanidad y Consumo, Spain
Barry McCormack	Southhampton University, United Kingdom
Alex McKinney	John Snow, Inc., USA
Narantuya Mend	Mongolian Foundation for Open Society, Mongolia
Lorena Mendoza	AVESP, Venezuela
Hugo Mercer	World Health Organization, Switzerland
Catherine Michaud	Harvard Center for Population and Development Studies, USA
Sarah Michael	Global Equity Initiative, Harvard University, USA

Anne Mills	London School of Hygiene & Tropical Medicine, United Kingdom
Mykhaylo Minakov	International Renaissance Foundation, Ukraine
Gilbert Mliga	Ministry of Health, Tanzania
Charles Mock	Harborview Medical Center, USA
David Molyneux	Liverpool School of Tropical Medicine: Lymphatic Filariasis Support Center, United Kingdom
Dominic Montagu	University of California at Berkeley, USA
Anne-Marie Moulin	Centre d'Études et de Documentation Economiques, Juridiques et Sociales, Egypt
Chakaya Muhwa	Kenya Medical Research Institute, Kenya
Fitzhugh Mullan	Project HOPE, USA
Olive Munjanja	Commonwealth Secretariat, Tanzania
William Muraskin	Queens College, USA
Ramses Naga	University of Lausane, Switzerland
Pat Naidoo	Global Equity Gauge Alliance, Health Equity, Uganda
Vinand Nantulya	The Global Fund to Fight AIDS, Tuberculosis & Malaria, Switzerland
Vasant Narasimhan	McKinsey & Co., USA
Sidney Ndeki	Centre of Educational Development in Health, Tanzania
Peter Ndumbe	University of Yaounde, Cameroon
Desire Ndushabandi	Ministry of Health, Rwanda
Victor Neufeld	McMaster University, Canada
Gustavo Nigenda	Mexican Health Foundation, Mexico
Volodymyr Nikitin	International Centre for Policy Studies, Ukraine
John Norcini	Foundation for Advancement of International Medical Education and Research, USA
Anders Nordstrom	World Health Organization, Switzerland
Jose Noronha	Sate University of Rio de Janeiro, Brazil
Mary Northridge	American Journal of Public Health, Columbia University, USA
Antoinette Ntuli	Health Link, South Africa
Paul Nunn	World Health Organization, Switzerland
Frank Nyonator	Ghana Health Service, Ghana
Aislinn O'Dwyer	West Lancashire Primary Care Trust, United Kingdom
Stephan Ochiel	Kenya Medical Association, Kenya
Kepha Ombacho	Kenya Ministry of Health, Kenya
Stjepan Oreskovic	Andrija Stamper School of Public Health, Croatia
Miquel Orozco	CIES–UNAN, Nicaragua
Judith Oulton	International Council of Nurses, Switzerland
Ariel Pablos-Mendez	World Health Organization, Switzerland

Randall Packard	The Johns Hopkins University, USA
Vicharn Panich	The Knowledge Management Institute, Thailand
Ok Pannenborg	World Bank, USA
Rosemarie Paul	Head of the Health Section of the Commonwealth Secretariat, United Kingdom
Margie Peden	World Health Organization, Switzerland
Eileen Petit-Mshana	World Health Organization, The Gambia
Verona Phillips	University of Western Cape: School of Public Health, South Africa
Ann Phoya	Ministry of Health and Population, Malawi
Nhan Le Phuong	The Atlantic Philanthropies, Viet Nam
Oscar Picazo	World Bank, USA
William Pick	The University of Witwatersrand, South Africa
Yogan Pillay	The Equity Project, South Africa
Paulina Pino	Universidad de Chile: Escuela de Salud Publica, Chile
Paul Plsek	Paul E. Plsek & Associates, Inc., USA
Kaja Põlluste	University of Tartu, Estonia
Wiput Poolchareon	Health Systems Research Institute, Thailand
Alex Preker	World Bank, USA
Dainius Puras	Vilnius University, Lithuania
Emilio Quevedo	Universidad Nacional de Colombia, Colombia
Geeta Rao Gupta	International Center for Research on Women, India
Mario Raviglione	World Health Organization, Switzerland
Srinath Reddy	Initiative for Cardiovascular Health Research in the Developing Countries, India
Laura Reichenbach	Harvard Center for Population and Development Studies, USA
Heide Richter-Airijoki	World Health Organization, Switzerland
Pia Rockhold	The Ministry of Foreign Affairs, Denmark
Wiwat Rojanapithayakor	Ministry of Public Health, Thailand
Laura Rose	World Bank, USA
Mark Rosenberg	Task Force for Child Survival and Development, USA
Patricia Rosenfield	Carnegie Corporation of New York, USA
Doris Rouse	RTI International, Global Health Technologies, USA
M. Rovere	Universidad de Bs As, Argentina
Julia Royall	National Institutes of Health, USA
Andrzej Rys	Jagiellonian University, Poland
Danielle Samalin	Robert F. Wagner School of Public Health, USA
David Sanders	University of the Western Cape, South Africa
Jay Satia	International Council on Management of Population Programs, Malaysia

Robert Scherpbier	World Health Organization: Stop TB Program, Switzerland
Anamaria Schindler	Ashoka-McKinsey Center for Social Entrepreneurship, Brazil
Bert Schreuder	KIT, The Netherlands
Anthony Seddoh	Ghana Health Service, Ghana
Nelson Sewankambo	Makerere University, Uganda
Nodira Sharipova	Bukhara State Medical Institute, Uzbekistan
Della Sherratt	World Health Organization, Switzerland
Sakai Shizu	Juntendo University Medical School: History of Medicine, Japan
Oscar Sierra	Universidad de Antioquia, Venezuela
Steven Simeons	OECD Social Policy Division/ Health Policy Unit, France
Noah Simmons	The Soros Foundation, USA
Jawaya Small	University of Cape Town, South Africa
Peter Smith	University of York, United Kingdom
Barbara Solarsh	University of Natal, South Africa
Giorgio Solimano	Universidad de Chile: Escuela de Salud Publica, Chile
Viorel Soltan	The Soros Foundation, Moldova
Nancy Spence	The Commonwealth Secretariat, United Kingdom
Ralph Stacey	University of Hertforshire, United Kingdom
Hilary Standing	Sussex University, Institute of Development Studies, United Kingdom
Barbara Stilwell	World Health Organization, Switzerland
Miriam Struchiner	LTC/NUTES, Universidade Federal do Rio de Janeiro, Brazil
Agus Suwandano	Ministry of Health, Indonesia
Simon Szreter	St. John's College, Cambridge, United Kingdom
Yves Talbot	University of Toronto, Canada
Martin Taylor	Department for International Development, United Kingdom
Steve Tollman	Indepth Africa, South Africa
Jurien Toonen	KIT, The Netherlands
Josette Troon	University of Amsterdam, The Netherlands
Alexander Tsyplakov	OSI Assistance Foundation, Public Health Programs, Uzbekistan
Victor Ursu	The Soros Foundation, Moldova
Wim van Leberghe	World Health Organization, Switzerland
Jackie Wahba	University of Southampton, United Kingdom
Brian Walker	Resilience Alliance, Australia
Damien Walker	University of Warwick, United Kingdom

Ian Walker	University of Warwick, United Kingdom
Regine Webster	Bill and Melinda Gates Foundation, USA
Jonathan Welch	Harvard Medical School, USA
Miriam Were	National AIDS Control Council, Kenya
Marijke Wijnroks	The Netherlands Ministry of Foreign Affairs, The Netherlands
Timothy Wilson	United Kingdom
Christiane Wiskow	International Labour Organization, Switzerland
Rony Zachariah	Médecins Sans Frontières, Luxembourg
Jabu Zulu	University of Western Cape: School of Public Health, South Africa
Pascal Zurn	World Health Organization, Switzerland